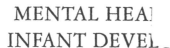

MENTAL HEAl
INFANT DEVEL

VOLUME TWO

Founded by C. K. Ogden

The International Library of Psychology

DEVELOPMENTAL PSYCHOLOGY
In 32 Volumes

MENTAL HEALTH AND INFANT DEVELOPMENT

Proceedings of the International Seminar held by the World Federation for Mental Health at Chichester, England

Volume Two: Case Histories

Edited by KENNETH SODDY

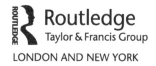

Routledge
Taylor & Francis Group

LONDON AND NEW YORK

First published 1955 by
Routledge and Kegan Paul Ltd.
Published 2013 by Routledge
2 Park Square, Milton Park, Abingdon, Oxfordshire OX14 4RN
711 Third Avenue, New York, NY 10017

First issued in paperback 2014

Routledge is an imprint of the Taylor and Francis Group, an informa business

British Library Cataloguing in Publication Data
A CIP catalogue record for this book
is available from the British Library

Mental Health and Infant Development
ISBN 0415-21008-9
Developmental Psychology: 32 Volumes
ISBN 0415-21128-X
The International Library of Psychology: 204 Volumes
ISBN 0415-19132-7

ISBN 978-1-138-87516-6 (pbk)
ISBN 978-0-415-21008-9 (hbk)

CONTENTS

EDITOR'S INTRODUCTION

EDITOR'S INTRODUCTION

THE PROCEEDINGS of the International Seminar on Mental Health and Infant Development, which was held by the World Federation for Mental Health at Bishop Otter College, Chichester, England, from 19th July to 10th August, 1952, have been published in two volumes, of which the present one constitutes the second. Volume I contains the lectures, and summaries of the discussions held during the Seminar; it includes also a description of the methods and techniques employed, and the reactions of the participants. From this account it can be seen that the Seminar constituted an important experiment in international, multi-professional, technical education in the field of mental health, and that the methods employed were also new in the international sphere.

Most short study courses make use only of the life experience and professional knowledge of those who are specially invited in order to instruct. At the Chichester Seminar, the basis of instruction was a series of case histories of living children, distributed in advance to all participants, for study before arrival. These individual case histories were supplemented by a number of sociological studies and films, some of which were specially prepared for the occasion. With a common library of factual material on which to base the study at the Seminar, the members of the Faculty were able, in addition to lecturing, to employ their experience and training in the illustration and enriching of the group discussions, by which method the Seminar mainly proceeded.

It has, unfortunately, not been possible to include, in this second Volume, all the material specially prepared for the Seminar. In order to keep it within reasonable proportions, and on account of the expense, we have been obliged to content ourselves with a representative sample of the case histories, selected roughly in proportion to the amount of preparatory material produced, respectively, in France, the United Kingdom, and the United States of America; but in addition to the collection of case histories, many special pieces of work were undertaken, and other material was provided, for the Seminar. The names of those who made themselves responsible for the provision of all this valuable material, and to whom grateful acknowledgment is due, are mentioned later in this introduction, while a list of the material itself is given at the end of it.

In France, a number of special studies were made of early childhood in a rural group, an urban artisan group and an 'intellectual'

3

group. Concurrently, studies were made of the relationship between parents' attitudes and the behaviour of young children in these three different cultural settings, and into the effects of social environments on the attitude of parents to children during infancy. The film of 'Monique', made under the direction of Dr. Jenny Aubry, was also available in an unfinished edition.

In the U.K., the case material was supplemented by an inquiry into child-rearing practices which had been carried out on a sample of mothers in an urban locality (Leeds), and the results of this questionnaire were available for study. In addition, a film entitled 'Life Begins in Leeds', directed by Mr. Arnold Joselin, was specially made for the occasion.

In the United States of America, also, many more individuals and institutions took part in the preparatory work than are represented by the case histories presented in this volume, and the Seminar was able to use films made by Dr. Margaret Fries, Dr. Margaret Mead and Mr. Gregory Bateson, Dr. René Spitz, and Professor Joseph Stone. Some of Dr. Spitz's film illustrations were specially prepared for the Seminar. Reference is made in Volume I to the use of this material.

The World Federation for Mental Health is greatly indebted to a large number of people whose activities made the Seminar possible and to whom due acknowledgment is paid in Volume I. Here I would like specially to refer to the grant of $15,000 made in August, 1951, by the United States Public Health Service to the Society for Applied Anthropology, for the preparation, under the direction of Dr. Margaret Mead, of case materials for use at the Seminar. The Seminar itself was held under the auspices of the World Federation for Mental Health in co-operation with the World Health Organization, UNESCO, the International Children's Centre in Paris, and the Grant Foundation of New York.

The intention, in collecting case materials, was to prepare a set of multi-professional case studies of individual children, to cover the period from conception to two years of age. The case studies were assembled from the existing records of institutions and of individuals engaged in child development research in the United States, and part of the funds was used to subsidize the collection of new case studies in France and the United Kingdom. The material was to include visual records, and samples of types of observation and records, and to illustrate their interpretation from the point of view of several professional disciplines. It was ultimately to be made generally available for teaching purposes, which is the intention of the present volume. For the Seminar itself, the material was provided in French and English.

The case histories from the United States included in this volume were contributed by the following institutions and personnel:

University of California Institute of Child Welfare: The Berkeley Growth Study and The Guidance Study, carried out by Dr. Harold E. Jones and Dr. Jean Macfarlane;

Fels Research Institute for the Study of Human Development, Antioch College, Yellow Springs, Ohio: Dr. L. W. Sontag;

Menninger Foundation, Topeka, Kansas: Dr. Sibylle Escalona (now at Child Study Centre, Yale University);

Departments of Psychiatry and Paediatrics, and the University Child Health Centre, University of Washington School of Medicine, Seattle, Washington: Dr. Ann H. Stewart, Dr. Charles A. Mangham, Dr. Herbert S. Ripley, Dr. Thomas H. Holmes and Dr. Robert W. Deisher;

Yale University School of Medicine: Dr. Ethelyn H. Klatskin, Miss Louise C. Wilkin, and Dr. Edith B. Jackson.

In France the collection of the case materials was under the general direction of Dr. Jenny Aubry, with the collaboration of Dr. Marcelle Geber, Dr. Cyrille Koupernik and Mme. Laurette Amado. Supplementary help in social ethnology was given by the Centre National de la Recherche Scientifique (Centre d'Etudes Sociologiques).

Field work was carried out in collaboration with representatives of the Laboratoire de Psychobiologie de l'Enfant, under Professor Henri Wallon, and the Institut de Biologie Sociale et d'Hygiène Mentale founded by Dr. Yves Porc'her.

The team of psychologists led by M. René Zazzo comprised Mme. Odette Brunet, Mlle. Irène Lézine, Mlle. Pierrette Brochay and Mme. Hilda Santucci. The team of ethnologists connected with the Centre d'Etudes Sociologiques and the Musée de l'Homme was led by M. P. Chombart de Lauwe and consisted of Dr. Geneviève Massé, Dr. Louis Massé, Mme. Marianne Le Guay and, for part of the time, M. J. Fournier.

Meetings for preparation and correlation were held under the chairmanship of Dr. Porc'her. The orientation and work method of the socio-ethnological research were those of M. Chombart de Lauwe.

In the United Kingdom the work of preparation of case material was under the direction of Professor D. R. MacCalman, Nuffield Professor of Psychiatry in the University of Leeds, with the co-operation of Professor G. P. Meredith, Professor of Psychology. Field work was carried out by members of the Departments of Psychiatry and Psychology, Mrs. Louise Mestel, Mrs. E. M. Stead, and Mr. Arnold Joselin, who directed the film. The work was carried through with the advice of a large and energetic inter-disciplinary committee drawn from the University and social agencies in the City.

It remains to record our gratitude to the parents and others who have so generously consented to allow the stories of their own and their children's lives to be reproduced for the benefit of students of child development throughout the world. All names and identifiable facts have been altered in order to preserve their anonymity, but it is possible that they may recognize themselves if these volumes should fall into their hands.

Grateful acknowledgments are due also to the staff of the World Federation for Mental Health, who were responsible for organizing the compilation, preparation and translation of all the documents, and particularly to Miss E. M. Thornton, the Secretary-General, for her help throughout, and especially in editing.

KENNETH SODDY, M.D.,

Assistant Director,
World Federation for Mental Health.

INTERNATIONAL SEMINAR ON MENTAL HEALTH AND INFANT DEVELOPMENT VOLUME II

Material specially provided for use at the Seminar, but not published in the Proceedings:—

UNITED STATES OF AMERICA

Case Histories

Tommy	Ruth
Jack	Felicia
Avis	Susan
Georgia	

Film Guides and Bibliographies

Anna	Abbey
Marie	Marvin
Helen	

FRANCE

Case Histories

The D. Family	The R. Family
The B. Family	The G. Family

Studies of Early Childhood

The Rural Group, by Pierrette Brochay and Louis Massé.

The Urban Industrial Group, by Odette Brunet and Marianne Le Guay.

The Group with Higher Education, by Irène Lézine, Louis Massé and Geneviève Massé.

Social Inquiries

Parents' Attitudes and the Behaviour of Young Children in Three Cultural Settings by René Zazzo and Hilda Santucci.

Social Environments and the Attitude of Parents to Children during Infancy by P. Chombart de Lauwe, with the collaboration of Louis and Geneviève Massé and Marianne Le Guay.

Observation and Treatment of a Case of Psychogenic Retardation—Monique, by Miriam David and Geneviève Appell.

UNITED KINGDOM

Case Histories

Charles
Andrew
Questionnaires to Mothers

7

INTRODUCTION TO THE STUDY OF
THE CASE HISTORIES

Margaret Mead

In this Volume we have brought together a selection from the case histories prepared in three countries by special teams, for use as teaching materials at the International Seminar on Mental Health and Infant Development, conducted by the World Federation for Mental Health at Chichester, England, in July and August, 1952.

We assembled these case histories because we felt that only by sharing concrete accounts of real children, in different societies, as seen through the eyes of members of several different professions and disciplines, could students of child development communicate with each other about problems of child care, education, and mental health. The particular composition of this group of case histories was determined by the situation within which the Seminar was conceived and executed, the decisions that the Faculty was to be multi-professional and tri-national, and that case materials should be assembled from the three countries represented on the Faculty, and presented in English and French. We also collected as much visual material as possible, and the Seminar itself made great use of films on infants and on child care (a list may be found in Vol. 1, p. 297); but for many of the case histories no film records were available. Some of the American studies date from a period before photography was much used in such studies; in other cases we could get good verbal records but no films. For the particular set of case histories presented here, we have no film record, but the cases have been organized to stand by themselves, so that they can be shared by any group of students or professional workers interested in studying child development.

There is great variety in the cases from the United States. They are drawn from many different parts of the country, and include studies of individuals who are now parents themselves; they vary from the rather slender observations on infants which were customary twenty-five years ago, to the most elaborate and detailed work of today. As the cases span twenty-five years, so also they span the whole period of changing child-care practice, from the rigid paediatric scheduling of the nineteen-twenties, to the newest practices of rooming-in[1] and self-regulation, of the nineteen-fifties.

The original selection of the cases proceeded by the following steps: a letter asking for co-operation was sent to those laboratories and individual research workers who might, a group of consultants thought, be willing to contribute material. They were requested, if possible, to present cases in pairs which showed some sort of contrast, with emphasis on the period from conception to the age of two. Ten laboratories and individuals co-operated, contributing eighteen cases, five of which were films with accompanying case descriptions.

From the remaining thirteen, six are presented here: *Fred*, who showed early difficulties but good later adjustment; *Cecilia*, showing good early adjustment, but difficulties in adolescence; *Bruce*, a child with pyloric stenosis who nevertheless made a good adjustment; *Sandra*, a child of only average endowment born to highly educated parents; *Joan*, the crying baby of a young near-psychotic veteran (ex-Service) father; and *Jerry*, a young, happy baby. Each of these cases was presented as one of a pair, except *Sandra*, which was one of a set of three, and *Bruce*, a case originally planned as one of a pair. A seventh case, *Felicia*, prepared by Dr. René Spitz, is referred to extensively in Volume I, as part of a lecture at the Seminar.

The cases are arranged from the eldest to the youngest, those covering the longer periods being designed to give perspective to the later cases in which only the very early years are available for study. In the first two cases a mass of material collected during periodic visits to the clinic is organized into an over-all description, while in the later cases the minute details of home visits and clinic visits are given. The student can thus obtain some feeling of the level of the inquiry, of the type of detail which is essential, and the way in which it can be organized into an over-all account.

All of the American cases have been presented so as to constitute a critical commentary on our present knowledge of the relationship between the needs and idiosyncratic constitution of the developing child, and current obstetric, paediatric and educational practices. They are more critical and less restricted to matters of fact than those from England and France. The contributors were very clearly oriented to the problems raised by changing practices, the details of which they gave. In the international setting of the Seminar, with an assumption that each nation might tend to emphasize the best in its practice, there was a risk that the amount of analytical self-criticisms in the material might be misunderstood: because the American

[1]'Rooming-in', a term derived from hospital Rooming-In Units, where mothers and new-born babies are housed together in private or semi-private rooms.

clinicians dwelt upon the defects in home or nursery, these might appear rather larger than life-size. It would be impossible to alter this self-searching critical emphasis without destroying the texture of the individual cases. It does, however, seem worth while to point out this danger in a publication which is planned for international use.

While the American contributors drew on already established, on-going studies, none of which were made especially for this collection, those from France and the United Kingdom were made specifically for the Seminar. The French studies were all made by the same team, all animated by the same point of view; contrast is provided by selecting cases from different social milieux—skilled urban industrial working-class, agricultural working-class, and an urban, highly educated group. In the French cases, although all are concerned with young children, the emphasis is on the whole family, the child in a family setting. In the American cases, on the other hand, the contrast lies in the methods and theoretical approaches used by the different research teams, while all of the children are of the middle-class, with the kind of parent who is willing to co-operate in this type of study. The five French cases presented here are selected from a group of nine; one other, the case of *Monique*, is described in Volume I, as part of Dr. Aubry's lecture. It is significant that in France it seems easier to get co-operation for a study such as this from working-class parents than from the middle-class. Extensive sociological survey work on child-rearing practices was undertaken in France also, and is reported in Volume I (Lézine).

The United Kingdom study was divided between a social survey of child-rearing practices, preparation of a film which showed the setting of childbirth in Leeds, and four case histories, of which those of two Jewish children, one regarded as normal, the other as needing clinical care, are presented here. The case histories were assembled in guided interviews which took note of the points which had also been included in a questionnaire, and are presented here under the questionnaire headings. The student is able to evaluate first the mother's responses to these questions, and then to read the summary of the cases as provided by the research group.

Interdisciplinary research of this sort has only been undertaken during the last twenty-five years, and owes its inspiration to the concept of the child as a whole person, about whom each discipline—the psychologist, psychiatrist, paediatrician, social worker, educator—is equipped to make professionally competent, but necessarily limited, judgements. By pooling their insights, a more complete concept of the child is obtained; through the individual child's uniqueness as a personality, these partial insights of several workers using different methods over a period of time, are organized into a meaningful whole. Parallel with research in child development, there grew up the idea of the child guidance team, again based on a recognition that different skills were needed if a child, especially a child in a home situation, in active relationship to parents and siblings, school-mates and teachers, was to receive proper help.

Since the first long-term studies were inaugurated over thirty years ago, the interdisciplinary teams and the children whom they have studied have grown together in knowledge of the intricacy and complexity of human growth. In the records, marking symbols have changed to sentences, sentences to paragraphs, paragraphs are now supplemented by films, and soon they will be supplemented by sound recordings. We have, in fact, come to recognize the existence of such matters as the way in which mother and child affect each other, the importance of the different sensory modalities in different children, the depth with which culture is represented in each, the patterning of behaviour, the varying amount of differentiation in the growth style of one child as compared with another, the extreme importance of the exact moment when—in the course of maturation—a bad event, a trauma, or a good event, a blessing, occurs. Interdisciplinary work has at times been very analytical, almost atomizing; at other times holistic. By its very nature such work must shift and change and alternate in emphases. The publication of these case histories and the discussions which they evoke, should themselves change the way in which interdisciplinary work in child development and child guidance is done tomorrow, and the day after.

In using these case histories for study, it will be essential to keep their design in mind. They are not intended to be studied separately by different members of a group. They are so designed that whether one or all are read, the cases used should be read and studied by the entire group which is to discuss them, so that difficulties of understanding, as between individuals of different temperament, different degrees of technical or theoretical knowledge, different theoretical orientation, different disciplinary practice, and different nationalities, can be bridged by references to '*Jerry's* mother', '*Joan's* crying fits', 'the housing problem of the French *L.* family', etc. These situations—*Jerry's* mother's way of amusing him, *Joan's* heartbroken crying in response to her mother's misery, the exigencies of four people living in one room—are described in words which necessarily carry different meanings to different people, but they are real people and real situations about which a good deal of meaningful detail has been assembled. This circumstance makes them more suitable for interdisciplinary study than formulations about 'anxiety', 'precocity', 'degree of verbalization', 'dependency', and all of the other verbal labels with which people who share one theoretical approach tend to communicate with each other. 'Cramped quarters' mean very different things in different countries, between different social levels; but in the description in the French cases, these different meanings are not permitted to obscure a point. We know just how many rooms there were, how they were arranged, who slept where, and how unusual this was for a given class. Terms like 'good heredity', 'a good family history', also come to life as the cases describe the actual occupation and reputed character of grandparents and great-grandparents. 'Response to parental strain' takes on meaning when, in a case like that of *Joan*, the reports of the father and mother on their sex relationships are correlated with records of the infant's crying.

Just as the concrete details about real people are designed to facilitate communication, so also we have tried, by the inclusion of facsimile and verbatim records, to give content to expressions such as 'the Rorschach protocol showed', 'behaviour at the physical examination indicated', 'the home visit suggested', 'a profile of the child showed normality'.

The inclusion of cases from three cultures, however much the methods of collection and analysis differed, will lead both towards a realization of the differences between cultures in major assumptions and in child-rearing practices, and a recognition that, in the western world, we are coming to share a common body of knowledge and practice about paediatrics and child care. The dangers as well as the advantages of this assumption that western medicine and western education are essentially one, all concerned with the currently demonstrable scientific truths, have to be borne in mind constantly, lest a practice deeply embedded in the culture of one country, be translated too heavily weighted with local cultural content, into another. (*See* Vol. I, p. 180). Continual cross-reference from the practice of one country to that of another, from *Danielle* to *Sandra* to *Charles*, from the housing of cold, foggy Leeds to the housing of California, serves as a reminder of the differences as well as the similarities between children reared in different parts of the western world. The explicit contrasts also provide useful documentation for representatives of the countries of Asia, of Africa and Oceania, who wish to discriminate between what is local and what may have more universal value.

Finally, it is important to realize that although we have called these papers 'case histories', because that is the tradition inherited from medicine, these are living children, human beings who, because their parents have co-operated in this scientific research, are making a unique and very much needed contribution to our knowledge of infancy and childhood. The student who uses these accounts may find it helpful to speak always as if the parents of the children were present, learning to deal with the characteristics that are presented here in somewhat formal, academic or clinical style, in such a way that they remain part of ordinary human intercourse. This should be the more useful an exercise in that the conventions of medicine and social research were developed before the full co-operation of human beings in professional work had been conceptualized, and case records too often retain the flavour of the charity ward and the medical demonstration. The parents of these children consented to their children's lives being turned into open books, not out of illness or necessity, but as a free gift to a questing world.

Part One

AMERICAN

CASE

HISTORIES

---

1. FRED

Twenty-three years old

INTRODUCTION

The case of Fred M. is taken from a longitudinal study of individuals from birth through twenty-one years and beyond. Each child was seen by appointment, near his birthday, once a month during infancy, then every three months until three years, and every six months through eighteen years. The observations included tests of mental and motor ability, anthropometric measurements, tests of development of reflexes and vegetative function, physical examinations, body photographs, X-rays of hand and knee, a series of personality and interest questionnaires, and ratings and notes on the child and his parents, as seen in the testing situation. In addition there were several interviews with the parents in the home, concerning family adjustments and attitudes. On the basis of home visits ratings were made of socio-economic status and other relevant aspects of the home and family.

The case history of Fred has been written after a careful reading through of all the test records, ratings, observations and interview material. It is presented as a running narrative of his development, in the setting of his home and family life as pieced together from the records.

CASE SUMMARY

Fred is now twenty-three. He enlisted in the army three years ago and since then he has gradually worked his way up to the rank of sergeant. His duties are mechanical and technical and have involved rather specialized training during his army career. From all reports Fred has developed interest and skill in his work, and now views his army training as preparation for mechanical work in civilian life. He was assigned his duties on the basis of army aptitude tests and apparently the assignment has turned out well. Successful enough to receive promotions, Fred is happy in his job and has been sought by his superiors to fill vacancies when they occurred. At one time Fred's parents were disappointed that he entered the army rather than continue his schooling, but now they are convinced that army training has helped him find what will probably be his niche in life.

Physically Fred is a very large young man. He is about two inches taller than six feet and weighs around 180 pounds. He has always been stronger than average, particularly in his left hand (he is left-handed),

17

and is now good-looking, with straight blond hair and blue eyes. Certainly his size should be an asset to him in the army, and, later, as a civilian. He stands erect, he is strong and solid, and he makes a good first impression, physically speaking.

Our most recent mental test information about Fred was gathered when he was eighteen. At that time his I.Q. was 112, and presumably it has not changed a great deal since then. Previous tests varied from 95 to 120, with little systematic trend over the years. Apparently Fred is intelligent enough to succeed in the army and in later life. His army aptitude tests were high enough for him to be selected for special training, and there is no reason to doubt that his intelligence is, if anything, slightly better than average, though he is certainly not particularly gifted.

For information about Fred's current emotional and personality status we are reduced almost entirely to inferences. What we know comes largely from conversations with his mother, who has seen him briefly from time to time during the last three years. In Mrs. M.'s opinion, her son is fairly well contented with his temporary army life. He likes the work and performs it successfully. He seems cheerful, though a little disturbed because the Korean war kept him in the army, and he is hopeful for the future. He has at least vague plans for his post-war life and is pleased that his army training gives promise of being useful to him later. He has already served overseas, though not in Korea, and is glad that he is unlikely to have to do so again. He is now entrusted with enough responsibility to make him feel worthwhile and useful, instead of a cog in a machine. Fred's personal and social adjustment are unknown and we have no information about his sexual adjustment. However, it seems reasonable to suppose that he is getting along no worse than average. His cheerfulness, his mildly hopeful optimism and his vocational success all suggest adequate functioning. Evidently army life and its new experiences agree with Fred; but whether his post-army life will continue to satisfy him, of course remains to be seen.

Mrs. M., the second of two girls, may well have been an unwanted child. Certainly she was unwanted by her older sister who teased her throughout much of her early childhood. Her father, a rather successful man, refused to help either daughter go to college and, according to Mrs. M.'s account, was a stern, cold, rigid task-master. There is no indication that he was brutal to his daughters, but coldness, lack of sympathy and affection can hardly be doubted. Mrs. M.'s mother, who died suddenly when her younger daughter was fourteen, was also a cold, unfriendly person. Mrs. M.'s account of her childhood reports maternal favouritism for the older sister, lack of emotional support and absence of any real love from her mother. How much of this interpretation is due to the parents themselves and how much is contributed by Mrs. M. is a little hard to ascertain. She admits to feeling no affection for either parent, and presumably her experiences as a child were responsible for this attitude.

After her mother's death Mrs. M. was given complete responsibility for managing her father's household. She reports bitter scenes with him about money, even though the money was there to be used for household needs, and views this period of her life as extremely unhappy. Her father's stinginess and refusal to help her led her to leave home when she was nineteen. She moved into an apartment with her sister and three years later she married. The circumstances which led to marriage have never been divulged to us, and both Mr. and Mrs. M. have shown reluctance to discuss the matter with interviewers.

Mr. M., like his wife, comes from German stock. He is a tall man who weighs 185 pounds, and he is ten years older than his wife. He was the second of several children and apparently suffered a good deal of brutality at the hands of his father. While Mr. M. seems not to have resented his father's physical beatings and frankly subscribes to the theory that 'to spare the rod is to spoil the child', Mrs. M. is extraordinarily vehement on the subject. In interviews and questionnaires during Fred's early childhood she was not content with mere comment about her own parents and childhood, but insisted that Mr. M. change the report about his. Evidently she did not wish to see her father-in-law put in a more kindly light than her own father, whom she regarded as a cold, disagreeable, and completely unsatisfactory parent. Mr. M. finally did so, but he continued to observe that a few good lickings[1] every so often were the only means by which boys could be kept disciplined. His own father considered women chattels, and his mother died in childbirth when he was nine years old. She had had seven children in nine years.

The M.s spent the first ten years of their marriage in the wide open spaces of the western United States. Mrs. M. reports that she was somewhat disturbed because she hadn't gone to college and might have done so then, but her status as the wife of a man in his thirties made the role of student incompatible to her. Her husband had not only finished college, but had a Master's degree as well. She admitted to misleading people for years about her educational achievements and avoided confessing the fact that she had never quite completed high school. During the ten years before Fred was born, life for the M.s was not perfect, and although Mrs. M. referred to the period as the 'gipsy days', she was not entirely happy about them. Left alone

---

[1]A colloquialism for a whipping, which may be moderately severe, but not so severe as a beating.

19

for weeks at a time while her husband was away on business, she found few friends and little entertainment in the small towns where they lived. Interviews with Mrs. M. reveal that while she looked back at the gay, romantic life of a 'gipsy' as foot-loose and carefree, it was also a time of loneliness and disappointment for her.

After ten years of marriage Mr. M.'s work transferred him to this community. His wife became pregnant almost immediately, much to their surprise. She reported shortly after Fred was born, that she had 'tried many different things' to become pregnant earlier in the marriage and had finally accepted the fact that she would have no children. Nothing in the very early records of Fred and his family suggest that he was an unwanted child. Nor does anything in the early records suggest that his birth was planned. We cannot doubt that the pregnancy was unsettling after ten years of marriage, since the foot-loose life with few responsibilities had to end. Mr. M. at forty-three had become accustomed to life without children, and his wife, who was thirty-three when Fred was born, said frequently that she was somewhat older than average when she had her first child. Whether they were pleased to have a baby at last, annoyed because their well-established routines were upset, or merely interested to see what parenthood was going to be like, is hard to say. One thing seems clear: during Fred's first year his mother was more anxious than the average mother. She worried about Fred's health, minor food dislikes, normal everyday events in his babyhood and the general question of child rearing, and mentioned that she had been concerned throughout pregnancy about the responsibility of caring for a baby. She was aware that she knew little or nothing about babies and wondered how she could manage. It seems reasonable to believe Mrs. M.'s report. How much else she thought can only be inferred, and it will be seen that her later behaviour makes it difficult to infer with certainty.

Regardless of what his parents may or may not have been thinking, pre-natal life was apparently normal for Fred. His mother visited the obstetrician once during the first month of pregnancy, twice each month thereafter until the eighth and ninth months when she made three visits. During pregnancy her health was good; except for slight nausea during the first months and œdema of the ankles during the last month, nothing untoward is reported. She gained twenty-nine pounds, her blood pressure, urine, and pelvic examinations were all normal. Although Mrs. M. experienced some mild discomfort during pregnancy, she was able to perform her household tasks throughout the entire period. She had a number of household appliances to make her work easier, and there is no indication of anything even remotely approximating difficulty or danger during pregnancy.

20

Fred was born at term, with delivery by breech presentation. Labour lasted fifteen hours. The arms were delivered easily, but there was some difficulty with the head. Deep episiotomy and laceration which included the anal sphincter were repaired during the period of hospitalization. Mrs. M. was allowed to sit up on the ninth day, and recovery continued satisfactorily. Fred was first observed in the hospital when he was three days old and appeared none the worse for his unusual style of birth. Heart rate, respiration, and infantile reflexes were normal. He weighed nine pounds ten ounces at birth, regained birth weight rapidly, and was ten pounds six ounces at one month. Fred was circumcised at the hospital and went home with his mother, when he was fourteen days old, to the family's modern three-room apartment. Theirs was a clean, neat, attractively furnished apartment with a southern exposure, and impressed us as being larger than average. The bathroom had both shower and tub, and Mrs. M. had for her use a vacuum-sweeper, electric mixer, washing-machine, and automatic water-heater. Fred spent much of his time during the first few months outdoors in the small garden and paved back-yard, both of which were easily accessible to the apartment.

Socio-economically, the family Fred was entering might be called middle middle-class American. Their income was $2,800 a year, somewhat above the current American mean. Mr. M., who had been employed by the government in outdoor conservation work during the first ten years of his marriage, was still a government employee, in a different job involving more desk work.

Fred was measured, weighed and tested every month for the first year. He progressed normally, gained weight each month, and on his first birthday weighed twenty-seven pounds four ounces. At that time he was thirty-two inches long, and his skeletal age was one year and three months. Even then Fred's systematic tendency toward slightly accelerated physical maturity was evident. In fact, at every age from the first to the seventeenth birthday, Fred was somewhat more mature skeletally than the average child of his age. This is especially true of his early childhood: at two years he was nine months in advance of the norms for his age, and at three he was fifteen months accelerated. This accelerated pattern of physical development was also noticeable in Fred's tooth eruption. His two lower front teeth appeared at five months, the upper two front teeth at seven and eight months, and by the time he was fifteen months old he had thirteen teeth.

Fred's early motor development was only slightly accelerated. He was able to sit alone when seven months old; crawling and creeping appeared toward the end of his ninth month, and by the end of the twelfth month he was able to take a few walking steps unaided. As

21

compared with his own physical development, Fred's motor development was not advanced, though it was a little superior to average development in the United States.

Fred was breast-fed for close to six months, though even in the hospital he had to have supplementary formula. Originally on a four-hour schedule, he was cut to five feedings a day by the time he was three months old. There is no record of when he was weaned from the bottle, though some time between twelve and fifteen months seems most likely. It was certainly accomplished without difficulty; neither then nor at any later period did Mrs. M. refer to it as a problem, though she constantly referred to his thumb-sucking.

Fred's diet became more varied as he grew older. Half an ounce of orange juice was added when he was three months old, by six months he was getting prune-pulp and apple-sauce along with cereal, a number of cooked vegetables and egg yolk. Bland desserts were included by nine months, and when he was a year old Fred had begun to eat raw fruit and some kinds of meat, though he did not like liver. Throughout his second and third years more and more foods were added. He was reported to be very fond of milk, eggs, meat, and fruit. Occasionally he seemed to reject a particular food for a brief period, but except for toast, none of the dislikes persisted for long. It was characteristic of him not to like coarse hard foods, particularly when they were first introduced. Otherwise nothing unusual can be found in Fred's food habits during the first three years.

So much then for Fred's earliest period. Pre-natally and hereditarily he seems to have got not worse than an average start in life, perhaps better than average. Except for a complicated birth and a mother somewhat older than most, very little in the way of difficulty can be anticipated from biological sources. Fred was a big baby, essentially normal at delivery, and from average to accelerated in physical, structural and motor development. Physically Fred has remained above average all his life, and his mental test scores have been average to above average.

Let us turn now to Fred's early environment and early personality development. When he was first brought to the clinic for measuring and testing, his mother impressed the staff as a competent, calm, mature, interested, and affectionate mother with a nice, handsome baby. He was rated 'happy', 'very happy', and 'extremely happy' during his tests the first year or so. Month after month the clinic noted him as being particularly responsive to social stimuli and very interested in the tests, the procedures, and the people he met. He cried infrequently and was one of the best-behaved babies in the study so far as fears, shyness and negativism were concerned. One would be inclined to say, if anything can be said about personality in

22

the first year of life, that Fred was developing easily, normally, and without difficulty.

To be sure, his development was not entirely smooth. As early as his first month his mother reported that he was sucking his thumb, and she was clearly concerned about it. During the first year Mrs. M. attempted many methods to prevent thumb-sucking, without result. She tied the sleeves of his nightclothes so that his hands couldn't extend through them, she tied the sleeves themselves to the sheets, and she bought aluminium mittens for him. She disapproved heartily of mothers who ignored thumb-sucking, and disagreed with her husband about the cause of the behaviour in Fred. Mr. M. was convinced that his son needed more food, and his wife consulted a dietician who assured her that his weight-gains indicated he was getting enough to eat. It seems unlikely that his early feeding was the source of the difficulty. He was breast-fed for the first four months of life and weaned gradually to the bottle. He took to the bottle well and continued to gain weight. Furthermore, Fred was sucking his thumb before he was a month old, when he was being breast-fed six times a day and before his early teething could have been responsible. It should be observed, too, that thumb-sucking seemed to be no problem to Fred (unless by definition the behaviour is said to be a symptom of tension), for he was a happy, contented, responsive baby. He was as well-behaved at home as he was on clinic visits, and both parents continually referred to his placidity, cheerfulness, and happy disposition. He seldom cried, and smiled a lot. He was, his mother claimed, easy to take care of and a pleasure both to her and her husband.

Aside from thumb-sucking, there is only one developmental anomaly in the first year. As early as the first month's visit Mrs. M. was concerned about Fred's constipation, and the concern continued throughout the first year. With and without physicians' advice she tried laxatives, diet change, and suppositories, without effect. Fred's bowel movements were infrequent, and as he grew older they averaged less than one a day. Mrs. M. fought a prolonged intermittent battle with Fred's physiological rhythms and the precise age at which she finally accepted them is not clear. Toilet-training was started when he was fourteen months old; his mother had previously remarked that she didn't mind changing and washing diapers. She had a washing-machine and observed that the amount of soil a baby produced seemed to her inconsequential.

When Fred was ten months old, Mrs. M. became aware that she was pregnant again. It is in the tenth month that we begin to find in the notes and records indications of a new side of Mrs. M.'s behaviour and feelings toward Fred. She reported then that Fred was more devoted to his father than to her, that his father was spoiling him by treating him as a plaything, and that his crying got on her nerves. He cried for attention in his father's absence, she explained, and she was left with the problem of curing the behaviour. What events might have occurred at this time to turn the child away from his mother and toward his father cannot be known. Nor can we tell how much of Mrs. M.'s report was coloured by her condition and how much by Fred's behaviour. During the clinic visit she appeared irritated by Fred, who cried several times and was scolded for it by his mother.

At eleven months Fred began to refuse food he didn't like and Mrs. M. decided that 'you have to kid them along to get them to eat what you want them to'. Her husband's approach to the problem differed. He scolded his son for not eating, and on one occasion, his wife reported, he hit Fred when he wouldn't eat what was offered him. This was the first indication we had that Mr. M. was assuming the role of disciplinarian, which he had previously avoided.

Apparently, once Fred became active, Mrs. M.'s problems and worries increased. He ate paper, put pebbles and matches in his mouth, persisted in trying to walk without support, which led to falls and bruises, and continued to cry for attention. Although she complained about the annoyance he caused her, she still seemed fond of Fred and was unwilling to place him in a nursery school because it would involve daily separation from him. She herself was obviously miserable in her pregnancy. Though she appeared to be in good health, her complaints were many, and she seemed to be trying to convince others, as well as herself, that she had serious symptoms.

When he was a year old Fred was sick from time to time, and the doctor diagnosed his trouble as the result of enlarged tonsils. His mother worried about him more than ever, gave in to his wishes and demands, and humoured him in his eating. She noticed about this time that Fred was definitely left-handed. At fourteen months toilet-training began, and at fifteen months Mrs. M. reported that Fred was more attached to his father than ever. Her appearance would start him yelling, she claimed, but he showed obvious delight whenever his father came home. This, she added, was despite the fact that his father forced him to do things she made no issue of and permitted him to get far more upset than she did.

On their eighteen months' visit to the clinic Mrs. M. was expecting her second baby to be born within a few days. She was tired, uncomfortable and nervous, and nagged Fred when he cried. Fred was still a feeding-problem and persisted in crying for attention.

When he saw clinic workers at twenty-one months his reactions showed a decided change. Abruptly, it seemed, he had become unresponsive to people, quite inactive and slow-moving, and uninterested

24

in toys. His physical condition was below par because of his enlarged tonsils, and his mother appeared more harried than ever with two children to care for. Mrs. M. claimed that Fred was very fond of his new brother, but neglected to mention that he had spat on the baby when he saw him for the first time. She recalled the incident considerably later. The care of two children she termed monotonous, and displayed none of the pleasure in them she showed when Fred was younger.

Fred had his tonsils out just before he was two, and his throat had healed completely by his clinic visit at twenty-four months. His mother said the tonsillectomy disturbed him not at all: certainly his general health had improved greatly. He was good-natured during the interview with clinic workers, but evidenced marked indifference for the first time toward testing. Mrs. M. reported that he was still his father's boy, and mentioned that she had been able to break Fred of handling his genitals, which she hadn't referred to previously. The behaviour bothered her because she was sure she kept him clean and observed no evidence of irritation. She punished him for it and resorted to slapping him when other punishment failed.

After Donald's birth, Mrs. M. seemed to be less critical of Fred who, at twenty-seven months, had learned to delight his parents with cute sounds and actions. At that age, however, and from that point on, the clinic reports of his visits noted consistent lack of interest, unresponsiveness and apathy in Fred. Although he could not be called unhappy, he was decidedly indifferent and antagonistic. At thirty months he displayed a tendency to do whatever he thought might attract scolding attention, and tried to have tasks performed for him, rather than perform them himself. He was restless and unco-operative, and Mrs. M. nagged him constantly. When he was fifty-four months old such behaviour was even more pronounced, and he had developed an attitude of passive resistance to all adult suggestions. By that time, too, he was a confirmed nail-biter. At five and a half years he impressed clinic workers by his failure to pay any attention to anything said to him, and at seven he made few verbal responses except 'I don't know' and 'I can't'.

From this point on in Fred's life he deteriorated to a low, unhappy, unsuccessful level. Throughout elementary school and high school his grades were poor. On one occasion he was held over a year in school to repeat the work. Another time he was doing so poorly and had made such a bad impression on his teachers that he was seriously considered as a candidate for special classes for feeble-minded and retarded children. He was taken out of one school and put into another. He attended a private school for a while where he improved, but not for long. Academically, Fred had become a dismal failure.

At home, during Fred's later childhood and adolescence, he fared little better. By the time he entered elementary school his parents had both come to view him as a disappointment and an annoyance. Mr. M.'s early fondness for his son disappeared. Instead he continually nagged him about his appearance, his table manners, his lack of success in school, his failure to pursue any useful hobby, his messy habits, and his generally unsatisfactory style of life. When an occasional teacher took an interest in Fred and suggested that he be encouraged to read, Mr. M. selected the books and forced Fred to read to him for one hour every evening. The books selected were interesting to Mr. M., rather than of interest to Fred. So Fred continued to be a poor reader in school and seldom read at home except when he was obliged to. The negativism thus induced in Fred simply compounded his difficulties. When it was discovered that his poor reading might be due to visual difficulties and glasses were purchased, he refused to wear them. There is no doubt that he needed them, but he would not co-operate.

Fred's personal difficulties were reflected in his behaviour at the clinic, and he became more and more reluctant to come for annual testing and measuring. Though his mother always was able to force him to come and frequently stated her willingness to do so, Fred himself ceased to show interest from the time he entered elementary school. At test after test throughout the ten years from six to sixteen, Fred was noted as arriving late, trying to defer his appointment, paying no attention to the mental tests, and giving the first answer that occurred to him. His aim on these occasions seemed to be to get the business over with. He would assert, often erroneously, that such-and-such was the right answer and refuse to consider other possibilities. It was impossible to motivate him. Even the personality and projective tests failed to interest him. He came, he put in his time, he submitted to the procedures, and he left.

It is interesting that during his first fifteen months when Fred was characteristically a happy and still-loved baby, his mental test scores for fifteen successive testings were found to correlate zero with a composite of his attitude toward the test situation (happiness, responsiveness, shyness, etc.). Thereafter, from age two to age nine, the correlation becomes ·64, his scores going down as his attitudes worsened. In other words, after two years of age, Fred's tested intelligence seems definitely to have suffered from his unhappy, unco-operative attitude. The testers always felt that Fred's scores would have been significantly higher had he made a normal effort to succeed in the tasks presented to him.

Listless, apathetic, uncommunicative, and unco-operative, Fred was a disappointment to his parents, a nuisance to his teachers, and a

26

sad, ineffectual, unhappy person to himself. The older he became the less we were able to draw him out. We know little of his adolescence, of his heterosexual interests, of his hopes or aspirations, or of the way he felt about himself and his environment. We are certain only that he was miserable, unsuccessful and resisting. Our last contact with him personally occurred when he was eighteen and about to finish high school. Since then our information has come from phone conversations with his parents.

What accounts for this serious and progressive decline in Fred? His first year, and even his second year, were good ones. To be sure, his was a breech birth; a sibling was born; he spent a night in the hospital; he was punished for handling his genitals; his mother tried hard to stop his thumb-sucking, and his parents were somewhat older than average when they had babies around. But these sorts of things have happened to many other children without ill effect, and at the time there was no evidence of ill effect on Fred. Even though Mrs. M. began to make complaining remarks about her husband and about Fred toward the end of his first year, he appeared to members of the staff who worked with him as a happy, responsive, normally-developing little boy. It is hard to believe that so young a person would store up frustrations without showing tension at the time. Be that as it may, there is information about Fred's parents that we gathered later which seems to bear on the course of Fred's later development.

When Fred was about ten, the workers undertook a rather intensive study of the family. At that time everyone was impressed with the intense and thinly-veiled hostility between Mr. and Mrs. M. She made constant, nagging attempts to get her husband interested in books and theories about child development and child care. Mr. M. would have none of it. He remained firm in his conviction that children needed a good licking from time to time. The more Mrs. M. insisted, the more her husband resisted. He thought modern theories of child rearing were frilly folderol, and querulously and unsuccessfully urged his wife to take an interest in economics and politics. Her response was to become not merely uninterested, but positively intolerant of such subjects.

The marital disagreements between the M.s extended to almost every area of their lives. Mrs. M. had definite plans for landscaping which she attempted to carry out by judicious planning and careful planting. After several weeks of inactivity her husband would go into the garden and without consulting her prune what she wanted left alone, uproot what she had been nurturing tenderly, and replant where she wanted an open vista. In household management Mrs. M. was an almost compulsive perfectionist, who refused family help because it did not meet her standards, but complained about the amount of work she had to do. When Mr. M.'s increasingly severe migraine headaches were the problem, he insisted that they were due to heredity and nothing could be done, while Mrs. M. berated him for not going to the doctor. If the headaches were bad Mr. M. moaned about the house, making life miserable for everyone, and prompted his wife to refer to him as her third child. There is no need to detail every instance of marital discord between the M.s. It was apparent to every observer and in every little routine of life. They disapproved of each other's relatives and incessantly referred to their inadequacies, in interviews. Their interests were different to begin with and became more so with time. Their failure to co-operate with one another was so extreme that Mr. M. planned the family vacations without consulting his wife or children. He was annoyed when they refused to fall in with his plans to drive about the country, and ultimately took it out on his wife by refusing her the use of the car, even though it usually remained in the garage.

In the follow-up when Fred was ten, and frequently thereafter, Mrs. M. remembered with great vehemence that she had never wanted any children, that Fred was unplanned, unwanted, a shock, a terrible annoyance, and an irritable, difficult baby. This report contrasts strongly with what she said when Fred was a baby and with our observations of him in infancy. What does it mean? Had Mrs. M. really tried to become pregnant before Fred was born, or was it fiction that she had? If she had tried, was her lack of success finally accepted and the childless style of life adopted without reservation, only to find it suddenly disappear? Had she never wanted children and concluded that she didn't have to worry about it, only to discover she was mistaken? (This seems unlikely, for she had a uterine anomaly corrected a few years before Fred was born.) If she didn't want children, why did she have another shortly after Fred was born and soon after she had told us she didn't plan any others? Did she think that Fred was a sort of chance phenomenon? Or did she find that babies were actually rather pleasant to have around and decide to try it again? We cannot know the answer for sure. The writer ventures what to him seems the most plausible accounting.

Regardless of the Ms' history, it seems inconceivable that they did not soon come to love Fred as a baby. Their comments about Fred, their behaviour toward the baby, and their early co-operation with the clinic staff all support this interpretation. Fred's development as an infant agrees. What accounts for their change? One thing is apparent: even in their early visits to us they showed mutual hostility. The reader will remember that Mrs. M. protested vigorously against Mr. M.'s description of his father. She persisted for months and finally obliged him to change his comments. Mrs. M. also showed ambivalence toward the first ten years of the marriage: at one time it was a 'gipsy life', and at others she was lonesome, abandoned in strange places, friendless, without a house to keep, and devoid of entertainment. Both the M.s were reluctant to discuss the details of their courtship and marriage. Their interests were different to start with, and one can imagine that Mrs. M. felt some envy of her husband's educational accomplishments. They had moved from place to place, forming no lasting ties and no sound affectional relationships with other people. As children both had endured abuse, intolerance, and motherlessness. Such people are not likely to take easily to new and intricate interpersonal complications in middle-age. While it is easy to love a 'good', quiet baby, it is not so easy to make the adjustments and sacrifices in daily routine that a small child requires. It is particularly difficult if the already established social relations are not satisfactory. When Fred was only seven months old, Mr. M. disparaged his wife's contention that she could be of some help to a neighbour who had just had a new baby.

The writer's hypothesis, then, is that as Fred grew from a placid, easy-to-take-care-of baby to a constantly changing and demanding young child, he became more and more difficult for his parents to adjust to. The adjustment was complicated by his mother's second pregnancy, but it doubtless would have been difficult without it. As Fred grew more responsive, he was used by his parents to express their hostility toward each other. His father spoiled him partly because he liked him and partly to annoy his wife. Mrs. M. was alternately indulgent and stern because sometimes she was too tired to maintain her standards, and at other times she could claim to be undoing the evil her husband had wrought. Mrs. M., at least, seems to have developed jealousy and to have resented the fact that the baby began to like his father better. With a new baby she ultimately transferred much of her former affection to it, and as her inconsistent and unfriendly treatment of Fred continued, he became such a problem that his father ceased to be fond of him. Each parent was able to blame the other for Fred's deficiencies; each found Fred less and less likeable; and each found the other more and more objectionable. With Fred's younger brother present as a standard, Fred could only suffer by comparison. Where once Mrs. M. had refused to be separated from Fred by nursery school, it was with a sigh of relief that both parents entered him a couple of years later.

The school and high-school years were passed in a disapproving, hostile, nagging, quarrelsome home. It was unsupportive, unpleasant and unsympathetic. The environment grew worse rather than better as Mr. and Mrs. M. grew farther apart and more fixed in their ways.

Alone, unwanted, objectionable and unhappy, Fred could hardly have developed otherwise. School, friends, amusement, and interests were unsatisfactory because his parents disapproved, because they failed to encourage him, or because they had not taught him the necessary social skills.

We do not know how Fred is faring now, but his parents begin to sound pleased with his achievements. Objectively, he is making good progress in the army. On his first visit home his mother was annoyed because he seemed to be home only to eat and sleep. On later furloughs he began to visit with them. The facts are not clear, but a plausible inference is that Fred has begun to find himself at last. Away from a completely unsatisfactory family, his intelligence, physique and appearance have finally been given a chance.

2. CECILIA

In her early twenties

INTRODUCTION

This case of Cecilia R. was selected for presentation from a cross-section sample of two hundred and fifty children who were studied from birth to maturity, because she made most of her life adaptations with less strain and fewer problems than most children in the group.

The selection of the items from the case record and the write-up here presented was done by a child psychologist who had no part in the study and who, therefore, was perhaps less biased (or differently biased) than the workers who knew her and her family intimately over a long period of time.

Something should be said about the purposes and the nature of the whole study, for what we obtain and report on any given child depends, of course, upon our research philosophy, our sample, and the kinds of data we secured.

The purposes were to find out the facts of development, physical, mental and personality, of a group of normal children, the problems, bafflements and satisfactions they meet in the process of growing up to be adults, and the problems, bafflements and satisfactions that confront their parents in the process.

Our basic philosophy was that, in order to understand the durable and characteristic patterns of behaviours, feelings and attitudes that we label personality, we need to know (i) what the growing organism is like structurally, or, in other words, what it has to adapt *with*; (ii) what it is stimulated or inhibited by in its physical, cultural and familial environment, in other words, what it has to adapt *to*; and (iii) the adaptive patterns, overt and covert (action, verbalization, thinking, fantasy and psychosomatic patterns) that become organized into a characteristic and idiosyncratic personality.

To these ends we secured cumulative anthropometrics, skeletal X-rays, body photographs and sensory acuitym easurements to appraise constitution and growth, and full health and nutritional records which caused temporary or permanent change in structural equipment. We secured systematic intelligence measures to indicate status and variability in functions, and records of interests, activities and skills. We secured detailed records of Cecilia's environment, especially of the interpersonal relationships within the home, in school and with her peers, the values and training procedures of her parents, sibs

31

and teachers. We secured an inventory of her changing and durable behaviours over a period of time, as reported by her family members, teachers and by herself. We studied her dreams, fantasies and projective protocols, her attitudes toward herself and others and the attitudes of others toward her. Because of the cumulative data on a group of growing children in their changing environments, we could compare her to herself at different ages, and to other children with similar and dissimilar constitutions, environments, life histories and adaptive patterns.

CASE SUMMARY

Cecilia is a happy, good-looking young mother in her early twenties. She has a well-proportioned feminine figure, a cheerful year-old daughter, and an attractive young husband whose prospects of material and economic success are better than average. The husband, a fine physical specimen and a high school and college athlete, now teaches and coaches athletics in a suburban high school. They live in a duplex,[1] which isn't quite what they want, but the current housing shortage forced them to take what they could get.

Cecilia met her future husband during her first year in college. Their engagement was announced early in her sophomore year at her college sorority, and they were married the following summer. Cecilia was twenty, her husband a little older. That fall, rather than continue in college, Cecilia went to work to help the new family get off to a good financial start, while George finished his remaining year of college and obtained his teaching credentials.

Since both Cecilia's parents had graduated from college and most of Cecilia's friends continued through college to graduate, her parents, particularly her mother, were upset about her decision to abandon her education, but they were able to see that there was economic sense in the arrangement.[2] Economics explained, too, why they moved in with George's parents for the first year, even as her mother had done. Cecilia's mother was disturbed by their decision, not because her home afforded an overlooked alternative for Cecilia and George, but because she felt herself somewhat superior to George's parents and felt rejected by the choice. In addition, the repetition of the situation of her own early married years reactivated her own anxieties.

After the husband finished college, he found a job with little trouble. His athletic prowess and reputation doubtless helped. He is

[1] An apartment occupying two floors.
[2] It is of interest to note that twice as many girls in this study graduated from college as their mothers. Cecilia clearly is not in line with the general educational trend.

well qualified for the career he has chosen: his athletic skills and interests make him well-liked by his adolescent students, and he is happy to be coaching.

Cecilia has taken to marriage as a small child takes to a mud pie. She is delighted with her baby, her parents are pleased, too. George is enthusiastic about his family, his job, which he takes very seriously, and about working with youngsters. The marriage is off to a good start. The couple give every promise of leading happy and useful lives.

What, from her early history, would we have predicted about Cecilia's adulthood? From her infancy and early childhood could we have foreseen what we find? Both parents agree that Cecilia was a planned and wanted baby. Her older brother was born two and a half years before she was, and he, too, was planned for and wanted. The first pregnancy was normal, with no complications, and carried to term. The same was true when Mrs. R. was carrying Cecilia. She gained thirty pounds during her second pregnancy; her heart, blood pressure, and urine specimens were all normal; labour was spontaneous and lasted ten hours; gas was administered as an anaesthetic; no instruments were used and Cecilia was born without difficulty in a private hospital attended by a physician. She weighed seven pounds seven ounces (her brother weighed five pounds five ounces). Cecilia's mother was thirty-four when she was born, but her age, which was somewhat older than the average, appears to have had no effect on the pregnancy.

Cecilia's pre-natal environment was untroubled, her heredity is clear. Neither physical nor mental abnormality is present in either side of the family. All her grandparents lived to be considerably older than the average life-span of Americans; they died in their seventies and eighties. Her father's family was ancestor-conscious and 'old American', claiming a number of moderately distinguished members. Cecilia's mother's family had not been established in the United States for nearly so long, but they were educated and successful people. The large, affectionate family circle is partly accounted for by a strong, old-world culture that one of Cecilia's maternal grandparents still fostered.

Biologically speaking, Cecilia began life with a running start. What about her environment? It is here that we observe a few handicaps.

Her only sib, a brother, Pete, who was two and a half years older and slow maturing, did not have the same serene personality as his sister. He had spent his first few years in a house dominated by Mr. R.'s mother and spinster sisters, and by the time Cecilia was born he had become a difficult child. Subjected to an inconsistent mixture of Watsonian scheduling, old-maidish indulgence and maternal confusion, he learned to scream because 'I get what I want when I do'. Over-active, troublesome and hard to manage, Pete was a continual worry to his mother. Fortunately Mr. R. recognized the problems Pete created and sympathized with his wife. When Cecilia was born they both agreed there would be no repetition of the mistakes they had made in raising their son, and they not only moved out of the father's family home but some thousand miles away.

Cecilia's physical environment during her first years was what might be termed slightly better than average American. The family rented a small, comfortable frame house in a neighbourhood of houses similar to it. As a baby Cecilia slept in her parents' room in a bed of her own. The house was heated and furnished adequately with overstuffed furniture, washing-machine and radio. The children played in their backyard or in neighbours' backyards, with moderate supervision and a host of playmates. By the time Cecilia was born the R.s had achieved financial independence and their income was slightly above average. Back debts had been paid and Mrs. R. was able to hire occasional household help.

Cecilia's first two years represent a model of normal, trouble-free development. Except for a two months' visit to paternal relatives when she was eight months old, she remained in one geographical environment and the exclusive responsibility of her mother. She was breast-fed every four hours for more than a year and supplementary bottle-feedings began at six months. She was offered orange juice at six weeks, vegetables at six months, cereals at seven months, egg when she was about a year old, and meat by the time she was twenty-one months. Her birth-weight of seven pounds seven ounces increased to nine pounds when she was a month old, to eighteen pounds at a year, and slightly more than twenty-five pounds when she was two. Her first teeth appeared at twelve months, and by the time she was two she had sixteen teeth and measured thirty-three and three quarter inches.

During her first six weeks Cecilia was somewhat constipated, and when she was eleven months old she vomited; otherwise her first two years were without problems. She had no colds, no colic, no eczema —no physical difficulties of any sort. She had no significant behavioural or psychological disturbances, never sucked her thumb, nor offered to bite other people.

Cecilia's bowel and bladder training began early and were emiently successful and without any evidence of emotional upset. On a visit at the age of six months her grandmother began taking her to the toilet when she seemed about to perform. By the time she was nine months old she had ceased wetting her clothing and at a year she no longer wet the bed. Cecilia's mother wasn't quite sure just when she no longer needed to toilet Cecilia during the night, but it was apparently long before she was twenty-one months old.

Very few traumatic events turn up in Cecilia's early childhood, but one possible instance occurred when she was a little less than a year old. While relatives were visiting and the family routine disturbed, Cecilia tried to get what she wanted by holding her breath until she was blue in the face. After three or four such attempts, her mother dashed cold water in her face (Mrs. R's mother had done that to her when she was a child), and the behaviour was never repeated. Except for this episode, Cecilia's infancy was calm. She showed no fears, no precocious interest in sex, no jealousy or hostility, little dependency, but certainly no over-determined independence. In her physical and mental examinations she was variously reported as 'interested', 'happy', 'cheerful', and 'alert'. Record forms on which it was possible to note either too much or too little important behaviour are filled in with negatives. Neither physicians nor psychologists were able to find anything to worry about.

Cecilia's first mental test was taken when she was just past twenty-one months old and her second three months later. On both occasions she scored about two and a half standard deviations above the mean for our group; in terms of I.Q. she scored between 135 and 140. Her response to the test situation was co-operative and interested, she seemed aware of what she could not do, and stated matter-of-factly, 'I can't', when given tasks too difficult for her.

In summarizing Cecilia's first two years we can say that she started life with good heredity and good health. Geographically speaking, her environment was also good, the family (untypically for our group) remaining in the same home from her early years to her marriage, and she maintained continuous friendships from her early pre-school years to her marriage, thus avoiding playmate discontinuities characteristic of most urban American children. She was healthy, contented and poised, and intellectually she was considerably above average. Perhaps some of the intellectual precocity was due to environmental influences as well as hereditary ones, for her mother read to her daily and gave her considerable attention.

Cecilia's social environment was not perfect. From some points of view, at least, the absence of her father for six or eight months of the year during the early formative period would be thought a serious liability, particularly since her maladjusted older brother remained the only other male of importance in the environment. Pete was not only tense, erratic and full of anxiety, but he showed signs of being specifically maladjusted toward his younger sister. Occasionally, when Cecilia was about two, he made slightly malicious references to her at the clinic, projecting many of his own difficulties on to Cecilia.

He accused her of being selfish, a fussy eater, and a poor sleeper. Yet Cecilia was none of these things and Pete was all of them. Even when Cecilia was two and Pete close to five he seemed to feel inferior to her. She was a co-operative, pleasant, happy child and he was an insecure, difficult, unhappy one. However, not all of Pete's projections were entirely motivated from within, since both parents shamed him on occasion by comparing him unfavourably with his little sister. But though Pete may have had a number of understandable reasons for acting as he did, his role as the major representative of maleness in the family might well have had later undesirable consequences in Cecilia. Furthermore, Cecilia's father was not pleased that his second child turned out to be a girl, and it wasn't until after Cecilia was two that he came to know and enjoy her. Until then he might have been called cool, if not actually rejecting.

A second source of possible difficulty for Cecilia was her parents' differences in temperament. Mr. R. was a sensible, emotionally unexpressive, intellectual person who said that he selected his wife because he thought she would make 'a good mother for my children'. It was he who instructed his wife in sexual matters by giving her a book to read before they were married. He verbalized his approach to sex as a strictly biologically and scientifically informed one. Reason and efficiency were his values. He was in the formal sense considerably better educated than his wife and had had graduate training in universities abroad. Mrs. R. was a warm, romantic, emotional woman who wept easily, as did her own mother, and thereby annoyed her husband. Where sex was biological for Mr. R., it was much more to his wife, who never became completely reconciled to her husband's failure to mix it with affection. Beyond that she felt that he failed to provide an outlet for her artistic interests and talents. Even when he was home Mr. R. seemed content to remain there reading while his wife continued her duties as mother and housekeeper. He was neither unkind nor cruel and in his own intellectual way he sympathized with his wife's need to enjoy herself. He did not, however, help her beyond giving advice.

Regardless of one's theoretical predilections, it is a fact that nowhere in Cecilia's first two years is there any sign that the environmental situation led to difficulty. Whether this is because her biological start was so good, because the environment was not disturbed enough, or because the effects did not appear until later, is, at least for the writer, problematical. Readers, perhaps, will form their own opinion from the rest of Cecilia's history.

Throughout the remainder of her pre-school years Cecilia's health continued good. She had many fewer children's diseases than average: mumps at two and a half, a bladder infection at three, a mild influenza at four and a half, and mild cases of chicken-pox and a whooping-cough when she was five and a half. Inspecting physicians found only one complaint: a slight dissatisfaction with her posture. Otherwise she was considered average to above average in health, nutrition, and motor behaviour. On her fifth birthday she was forty-two and a half inches tall and weighed thirty-nine pounds. Her eyes, ears, teeth, lungs, heart, throat, skin, finger-nails, arms, legs—everything about her was in good condition.

On five mental tests between two and five years Cecilia was consistently scoring I.Q.s between 135 and 155. She showed marked verbal proficiency on all occasions, and although she remembered test items from one testing to the next, she displayed obvious interest.

Throughout her pre-school years, Cecilia's personality remained strong, without fears, anxieties, nervous habits, hostility, or dependency. She continued to be characterized as cheerful, friendly, alert, interested, co-operative and independent. She got along well with other children and even with Pete, whose jealousy and hostility diminished. Pete came to depend on Cecilia for support when troubled by night terrors, school problems and social disapproval. His need to be dependent unquestionably increased her self-confidence. Mrs. R. reported that Cecilia was easy to manage throughout the pre-school years, lost her temper not more than once a month and regained it quickly, without prolonged upset. She suspected that Cecilia's few outbursts were primarily imitative of Pete, who continued to be difficult and whose temper tantrums were now supplemented by night terrors and almost hallucinatory episodes. His infantile thumb-sucking had ceased, but he was now a confirmed nail-biter.

Throughout this period Cecilia showed increasing fondness for Pete. His difficulties did not estrange her from him, and she showed great sorrow and concern when he was scolded or reprimanded. This was despite the fact that Cecilia's father was away from home most of the time and took greater delight in playing masculine games with his son when he was home than in paying attention to his daughter. Mr. R. was not unkind to Cecilia but seemed more interested and sympathetic towards his son than towards her. Had Cecilia been a less sturdy organism she might well have taken her father's favouritism badly, but her mother continued to be placid, understanding, devoted and attentive to her children. She read to them daily and tried to help them in their play with neighbourhood friends. Mrs. R. was gradually becoming used to her husband's cool, intellectual style of life and expressed considerable gratitude for the help the clinic had given her in understanding him, herself and her children.

When Cecilia was thirty-six months old her mother told her that babies grew from a seed inside the mother and Cecilia accepted the fact with equanimity. She had been aware of anatomical differences between the sexes since she was a baby, and felt no concern about them. When she was four and a half she developed an unexpected degree of modesty around her brother, which presumably began as a result of some disapproved exhibitionistic sex play between Cecilia and another girl. This modesty persisted for a year or so and then disappeared without any specific action being taken.

Two other episodes related to Cecilia's psycho-sexual development occurred during the pre-school years. When she was four and a half she observed to a neighbour who had just had a baby girl but wanted a boy: 'If you really want a boy you should wish for a girl, and if you really want a girl you should wish for a boy. You always get the opposite of what you wish for.'

About the same time Cecilia remarked frequently to adults that when she grew up she wanted to be a married woman and that she would marry her father after her mother died. At the same time Cecilia was saying this she also said to her father: 'Boys should sleep with boys and girls should sleep with girls'. This rule she repeated to her father almost daily for a period of several months. Did it stem from guilt or simply from the fact that her father shooed her back to her own bed whenever she tried to crawl into bed with her mother? Both Cecilia and her mother enjoyed being in bed together in the morning during the months Mr. R. was away from home, and his return interrupted this.

This, then, was Cecilia when she started school: an extremely intelligent child with exceptionally good health, an attractive, integrated personality, and almost no symptoms of conflict. Except for the bizarre behaviour, anxiety and immaturity of her brother and the cool intellectuality of her father, she was subjected to insignificant environmental and biological stress during her infancy and early childhood. One is tempted to conclude that her early and successful adoption of the role of a young adult woman reflects the stability and consistency of her first years and to surmise that the passive acceptance and placidity which her mother showed toward her father made it possible for her to fill her adult role so easily. Certainly no one would doubt that her good start in life was a great help to her.

But what of the fifteen years between Cecilia's beginning school and her marriage? Had they no important effect on her? Why did she show so little interest in her education that she discontinued it, despite strong parental pressure to finish college and the great American push in that direction? Why did Cecilia choose a big, strong, prototypically successful college athlete for a husband, rather

38

than a man more like her small-sized, intellectual and reserved father or her small and tense brother? If the first few years are so important, why is it that Cecilia easily established rapport with big, almost stereotypical college males? She certainly had different kinds of males around her when she was a little girl. These, it seems to me, are legitimate questions. The answers will not be forthcoming in any complete sense, but a brief examination of the rest of Cecilia's history will be illuminating.

During kindergarten and the early grades Cecilia retained the popularity among children and adults alike, which had marked her pre-school years. Teachers called her 'an ideal child' and 'a privilege to teach', and a third of her third grade classmates called her their best friend. She was good at games, showed special talent in art, and her grades increased from good to excellent. Though they admired her and desired her friendship, Cecilia's schoolmates characterized her as 'bossy', but they were eager to add that she was a 'good sport', 'popular' and 'good looking'.

Cecilia's popularity increased and by the time she reached sixth grade she was known as 'good-looking', 'well-groomed', 'friendly', and a 'leader'. Her parents were proud of her, her teachers devoted to her, and one-fourth of her class still claimed her as their best friend. Her grades were still excellent, but during the sixth grade period she seemed to clinic workers to have lost much of her spontaneity and warmth. Weariness and determination replaced the zest and radiance she had displayed all her life.

At twelve Cecilia entered a large junior high school where her reputation for popularity flourished and she made many more friends. Her new teachers regarded her as highly as her elementary school teachers had, but one who had taught her previously noted that she seemed anxious and that her grades now included as many 'B's as 'A's. Cecilia worried about the 'B's and her mother felt that she was not living up to her expectations as the 'perfect' daughter.

In the eighth grade at thirteen, Cecilia was still the most popular member of her class. She had four 'best friends', her grades were once more all 'A's, and she had lost the tenseness and anxiety of the previous year. She was companionable, if detached, in her relationship with her family, and she began to display the quiet confidence of an adult.

Cecilia's physiological habits during this period were the result of normal development, good health, and a good regimen. She slept and ate well and elimination was never a problem. By six or seven years she demanded bathroom privacy but never showed embarrassment during physical examinations. The functions of the body were explained to her by both parents and she learned about procreation and menstruation at an early age. She also learned what was suitable to discuss once she had the factual information, after neighbourhood disapproval attended two attempts to share her knowledge with her playmates. Cecilia regarded her first menstruation at twelve as a symbol of maturity and it pleased her, though the eight months before and six months after its onset corresponded with her tense, toneless period. At thirteen she was less demonstrative towards her mother than she had been until then, but companionship with her father increased. Boys said she was good looking and her interest in them and attitude towards them were normal and healthy. When asked if she intended to marry and have children, she said she worried about finding a husband who would be fond of her but not let her dominate him. Because the boys at school were far less mature than she, she thought at thirteen that she might not marry—she would have no respect for a man who would be 'argued down' easily, and her ability to manage her male classmates discouraged her. She wanted children, but said she wouldn't think of marrying a man to have children because 'it wouldn't be fair to him'.

Cecilia's later childhood does not support the notion that she accepted from the beginning the docile, well-loved-woman's role. In fact it is quite clear that as she was entering adolescence she would have none of it. Her mother's passive role was not for her, and throughout adolescence we find the same theme repeated: she is concerned about dominance and will not be pushed around by either men or women, boys or girls. In many interviews during her adolescence she reiterated her interest in tall, large males, but in males whom she could not control, psychologically speaking. Occasionally she reported enjoyment of the physical strength of boys and men, but her major preoccupation was with the social, rather than the physical, aspects of dominance. She emphasized her desire for mature males, for she was an early-maturing girl. Though she often found herself in the role of a protective person with boys, and her older brother and some of her earlier boy friends were extremely dependent upon her, she never fully accepted a dominant role with them. It was only with mature males that she really enjoyed herself, and, although she was pleasant to boys whose social and intellectual superior she was, she never developed an intense interest in them.

During later adolescence Cecilia's social behaviour toward boys became complicated by Mrs. R.'s nagging, self-derogatory, regressive, menopausal dependence. Cecilia's mother made a dreadful nuisance of herself, whining, complaining and harrying Cecilia about her boy friends. The more mature the boy, the greater the maternal objection. She complained to her husband about Cecilia, and invoked Cecilia's wrath at what she termed her mother's 'nasty, dirty mind'.

At the same time Cecilia's grades in high school began to deteriorate. Unhappy at home, in the process of trying to emancipate herself as an adult, unable to find many boys of interest to her, and with integrity and intelligence enough to be dissatisfied with childish admiration from less mature youngsters, Cecilia spent a miserable couple of years. She understood her mother's personality extremely well and ultimately learned to manage her with great success. Her mother's dependency on her daughter's judgment added to Cecilia's confidence in herself. She became engaged after a year in college, where at last she met many big, intelligent, mature men, and after enjoying an academic year in the romantic status of an engaged sorority girl, she married and set to work to give her marriage financial and social security.

Readers may wish to interpret Cecilia's history according to their own theoretical positions. The writer suggests a commonsense one, not with the expectation that others will agree, but in the hope that discussants will find it a useful common reference point—even if only as something to attack.

Cecilia began life with superior biological and intellectual equipment. Her early years were almost entirely regulated by a kind, affectionate and devoted mother who started her out easily toward good mental health, socially acceptable habits and traits, and releases through art, music and reading. A rapid and easy learner, Cecilia developed intellectually and socially in superior fashion. Stable and intelligent, subjected to a consistent régime, Cecilia had little reason to develop problems. With strong emotional support from her mother and her playmates and no active rejection from her usually absent father, Cecilia felt secure during her first five years. No emotional discontinuities occurred save those due to her father's absence and some separation from her mother on his return. Her modesty about her body and her insistence that boys should sleep with boys, and girls with girls, seems to require no recondite explanation. The former seems no more than a simple and direct response to social disapproval that ultimately became desensitized. The latter represents an attempt to regain the cosy and affectionate pleasure she enjoyed with her mother.

The continuing good adjustment in elementary school requires little explanation. The difficulties in high school arose from two sources: the fact that Cecilia was an early-maturing girl of high intelligence who developed heterosexual interests that ran into maternal objection; and the fact that in the American educational system there is little opportunity for early-maturing girls to find boys who are their social and emotional equals. For Cecilia the difficulty was compounded by her intellectual superiority. As soon as she entered the large social environment of a big co-educational university, her social problems vanished. Alert to the cultural standards of her time, she chose the cultural ideal for a husband and put her intelligence to work building a happy and stable American marriage.

Cecilia's concern with dominance can most easily be traced to her mother's refusal to allow her to continue her normal, but perhaps precocious, development. Intelligent as she was, she wanted nothing to do with being the docile, maternal door-mat her mother had been. American emphasis on the equality of women was not lost on Cecilia. Mrs. R.'s conception of the role of a woman came from her mother and old-world traditions. Cecilia's came from American culture. Had her mother been a happier person in Cecilia's adolescence it is possible that Mrs. R.'s pattern would have seemed more attractive to her daughter; and while not following the door-mat pattern she got satisfaction making adaptations to her husband and chose one whom, at least on a physical basis, she couldn't dominate.

One loose end remains. Why, if Cecilia was intelligent and responsive to the social values of American society, did she fail to finish her college education? Perhaps her mother's educational status was not lost on Cecilia; or perhaps Cecilia's academic difficulties in high school had affected her attitude towards the scholastic. Perhaps the dammed-up interest in social maturity made achievement of full adult female status particularly desirable; or it may be that Cecilia was correct in her decision that the way to material and social success in an America of increasing income taxes requires the economic participation of both partners in a marriage. Or perhaps, after life-long social success and managerial skills in inter-personal relations, it was a relief to 'make the sacrifices', or maybe this was a disguised way of following her mother's patterns.

3. BRUCE
Eight years old

INTRODUCTION

The case of Bruce J. is taken from a longitudinal multidisciplined study of individuals from before birth to maturity. A research staff upon which many disciplines are represented studies the same children at frequent intervals, measuring many aspects of growth, maturation, and environment at different sequential developmental levels. The study is designed to produce a better understanding of various individual patterns of growth and maturation, and to further knowledge of the inter-relationships of such patterns and of the factors which may modify them. Some of the more important factors measured are:—

(i) The health, nutrition, and body chemistry of the mother during pregnancy.

(ii) The nature and level of foetal activity. (There is evidence that pre-natal patterns are predictive of post-natal activity patterns.)

(iii) Background materials, including mental tests, personality inventories, psychiatric histories, etc., of parents.

On the child, the data gathered include:

(i) *physical structure* as described by anthropometric methods, X-rays of soft tissue, skeleton;

(ii) *health* as measured by medical history, X-rays of chest, sinuses, etc., and physical examination;

(iii) *nutrition*, as determined from diet records and blood assays of some of the vitamins;

(iv) *endocrine function*, as determined from physical examination, enzyme and hormone assays;

(v) *mental growth*, as measured by a variety of tests;

(vi) *personality formation*, as determined by assessments of the emotional devices and defences of the child, his group adjustment, etc., and involving the use of group observations, ratings, projective techniques, and interviews;

(vii) *autonomic nervous system function*, as determined by a battery of tests involving measures of blood flow, blood pressure, skin temperature, heart rate, and skin conductance;

(viii) *environment*, in terms of type of community, structure and composition of the home, parental attitudes, schools, etc.

D
43

The products of the research staff consist of scientific papers dealing with various problems of development and function, and case material such as this one. Such cases are used both for the development and later testing of hypotheses, and as illustrative material for teaching purposes.

Instead of the usual chronological narrative, this case has been handled in the following manner:

First, a summary of what seem to the research staff to be the particularly interesting and significant aspects of the case.

Second, the actual clinical records—or abstracts taken from the clinical records—with which the research staff worked and upon which the summary is based. These medical, psychological, and observational data have been grouped under two general headings: Bruce's family, and Bruce himself.

CASE SUMMARY

Bruce J. is the elder son of a middle-class American family, his father aged 41, his mother aged 36. Both Mr. and Mrs. J. are fourth generation folk of English-Scotch-Irish origin. They are both Protestants and good church-goers. Both have high school educations. Mr. J. is a salesman, whose annual income before taxes is from $4,500 to $5,000 a year. The family is fairly representative of the middle-class population of this community, in which the population is almost entirely 'old American'. There has been no important European immigration here for many generations. Bruce has a younger brother, David, born when Bruce was 2 years and 4 months old.

The case of Bruce J. has been selected for presentation because, on the basis of certain aspects of his mother's environment and of his own development, one might well have predicted severe problems of behaviour and adjustment. Yet such problems have not only appeared only in a mild form, but seem to be well on the way toward resolution. The case illustrates very well certain psychosomatic and perhaps somatopsychic problems and how they may be important through their effect in modifying the child's environment. The term psychosomatic is most commonly used to describe certain kinds of dysfunction or illness in which an emotional factor is presumed to be, at least in part, of aetiological consequence. Such a use of the term fails to imply another psychosomatic, or preferably, somatopsychic relationship, namely, the way in which a physical disturbance, regardless of origin, may modify the environment and often the whole system of ego defences of the individual. For example, the child with a severe case of asthma may have that affliction in part because of an inadequate handling of infantile dependent love-needs, in turn, the

44

result of an aberrant feeling and behaviour pattern on the part of his mother. At the same time, his illness may modify his environment and it may, and almost certainly will, cause changes in his relationship to his mother and in his mother's behaviour toward him. Some of these changes are likely to be:

(i) The creation of over-solicitousness on the mother's part.
(ii) Increased repression of any hostilities she may have for her child.
(iii) Accentuation of hostility feelings even though they cannot be expressed (a less desirable, more demanding child).
(iv) Greater actual physical dependency of the child.
(v) Accentuation of guilt for hostility.

Certain aspects of Mrs. J.'s (Bruce's mother's) personality dynamics are of importance in her relationship to her child. Mrs. J. is the oldest of five children. Her father is a passive man who took little responsibility for discipline in the family, which was strongly dominated by his wife. He had a recurrent peptic ulcer which troubled him for a good many years of his life. Mrs. J.'s mother was a somewhat irascible and strongly-controlling woman in whose relationship to her children there was always a good deal of hostility. She offered a very difficult figure to her daughters for feminine identification—a fact which, together with the withdrawn and passive role of the father, might have been expected to create problems both of dependency and femininity in Mrs. J. When Mrs. J. was 18, her mother selected for her the man she was to marry. Mrs. J. rebelled at this, broke with her mother, and left home. Shortly thereafter she married a man of her own selection.

The intensity of her need for a home and family of her own may in some part result from these anxieties about dependency and femininity. Her high anxiety level existing for years, she herself associated with her feelings of hostility toward her mother. Mrs. J. suffered a stomach disturbance some years ago which was diagnosed as peptic ulcer and was perhaps related to her handling of her dependent needs. The anxiety level in this woman could be anticipated to be an important factor in her relationship to any children she might bear.

Her intense desire for a family was thrice frustrated in the first five years of her marriage by three miscarriages, cause unknown. She emerged from these experiences with a considerably heightened anxiety, but without any admitted concern about her ability to carry through to term the product of her fourth conception. She anticipated no trouble whatever, despite her history of miscarriages. Her calmness and tranquillity emphasize the importance of denial as one of her cardinal defences.

The pregnancy from which Bruce was born was uneventful, as was the labour. The presumed apprehension over the three miscarriages, coupled with the intensity of her desire to raise a large family, could well be expected to produce an over-protective and anxious relationship with the new-born child. Very shortly after birth, it became evident that Bruce could retain only a tiny portion of his feedings. The cause of his consistent regurgitation was diagnosed as congenital pyloric stenosis, and an early operation was done. These events might have been expected to increase the mother's apprehension immensely and to accentuate her over-protection. Her anxiety level was, of course, greatly heightened as a result of these events, but neither from the experiences with miscarriages nor the pyloric stenosis did there result the persistent and powerful pattern of over-protection which we anticipated. The somatopsychic effects of both the miscarriages and Bruce's pyloric stenosis are apparent in a heightened anxiety level which Bruce exhibits in certain situations at forty-two and forty-eight months. His slightly deviant nursery school behaviour in terms of peer relationships might be presumed to result from paternal relationship. On the other hand, his nursery school behaviour does not include anxiety about leaving home or excessive turning to teacher for help and reassurance, factors which we should expect in the child of over-protective parents whose response was not strongly aggressive and rebellious. Bruce's nursery school behaviour does show elements of aggression, but not at all at a level at which it might be looked upon as a powerful and neurotic defence. He has, on the other hand, certain fairly appropriate devices (his smiles, his persistent approach to his peers) for gaining peer acceptance and he seems to employ them without excessive anxiety.

It is of interest to know also that while it is possible that some of Bruce's behaviour (just described) may result in part from sibling rivalry with younger brother David, there is no evidence that this sibling rivalry is severe or has caused undue trouble. It is our feeling that the combination of the very strong mother-love, together with an extremely sensible expression of that love and programme for handling Bruce, which are characteristic of Mrs. J.'s family rearing, are responsible for this fact. This case illustrates well some of the difficulties of predicting behaviour patterns from the occurrence of what would be universally considered to be traumatic experiences.

It is of interest to know that in Bruce's family history, Bruce's maternal grandfather suffered from verified peptic ulcer, Bruce's mother suffered from verified peptic ulcer, Bruce's father has a verified peptic ulcer, and Bruce has a congenitally hypertrophied pylorus. Obviously this fact must be looked upon purely as a coincidence, yet an interesting one, for a realistic approach to the question of the

46

genetics of psychosomatic disorders must include the question of con-stitutional predisposition as well as the psychogenic factor.

RECORDS OF BRUCE'S FAMILY

(a) Family History

Child's Name—Bruce J. Birth Date, 3rd June, 1943.

FATHER: Name: Harry J.
Education: high school.
Married: 1935, age 29 years.
Occupation: owner of clothing store.
General health: fair, had ulcerated stomach in 1936.

FATHER'S FAMILY:
Father died at age 65, from T.B.
Occupation: farmer.
Health: ill for five years before death.
Mother—living (1942), 60 years old.
Occupation: housewife.
Health: good.
Siblings: one older brother living (1942), married, in good health.

MOTHER: Name: Helen J.
Education: high school.
Married: 1935, age 22.
Occupation: housewife. Worked as book-keeper for four years before marriage.
General health: Generally good. Had stomach ulcer, January, 1943: lost weight, very thin. Treatment taken and ulcer cleared up in July, 1947. Feeling well since.
Miscarriage—January, 1936.
Still-born—December, 1939.
Miscarriage—May, 1941.
First normal pregnancy (Bruce), 3rd June, 1943.
Second normal pregnancy (David), 3rd October, 1945.

MOTHER'S FAMILY:
Father died (1937) age 62, from high blood pressure.
Occupation: welder.
Health: in poor health for several years before death.

Mother living (1942), 58 years old.

Occupation: housewife.

Siblings: one younger brother: died at 20 years from leucaemia.

one younger brother living (1942), married, in good health; salesman.

one younger brother living (1942), married, in good health; in army.

one younger sister living (1942), married, in good health; housewife.

FAMILY DISEASE HISTORY

Tuberculosis:

Paternal grandfather died from T.B.

Ulcers:

Father and mother had stomach ulcers.

Heart trouble:

Maternal grandfather died from high blood pressure.

Leucaemia:

Maternal uncle died from leucaemia at 20 years of age.

(b) *Interviews with Mrs. J.*

(i) This interview took place on 15th December, 1944, when Bruce was just over 18 months old. The interviewer's notes were as follows:

Mrs. J. is one of a family of five: three boys, two girls. She is the oldest (33).

Married at 22; Bruce is the fourth pregnancy.

Mrs. J. was brought up on a farm. Had little responsibility for younger sibs. Her father is easy-going and voices little opinion; mother is more quick-tempered. Her mother tried to select a husband for Mrs. J. Mrs. J. is quite hostile to mother and has been for some time. She is weeping repeatedly in this interview. Hostility is heavily toward mother. My impression is that Mr. J. is the more dependent one.

Mrs. J. worked for four years after high school; has worked most of married life. Loves to care for children.

Had a major rebellion at 18 because of her mother's control and attempt to select husband. Considerable social relationships. Husband is punctual and orderly, 'I annoy him by being late'.

He corrects wife's language and irritates her. Had anxiety period in 1940 and 1941; was supposed to have peptic ulcer and 'nerves'. 'I've been more nervous since an operation in September'.

Has been fatigued, and had a terrible time dispelling the idea that the baby was only a dream. She traces anxiety to rebellion at time of marriage.

This woman has denied her dependent need of her mother; switched to Mr. J. and he doesn't measure up, so her dependent needs are not met and she is anxious.

(ii) This interview took place when Bruce was 24½ months old. Dated 15th June, 1945, the record reads:

Mrs. J. has become pregnant again and expects the new baby to be delivered on 10th October, 1945. Mrs. J. is delighted with the anticipated event and apparently has no apprehension whatever either about the possibility of another miscarriage or about Bruce's acceptance of the new baby. This was a planned pregnancy.

(c) Interpretations of Mrs. J.'s Projective Tests

Mrs. J. was given three standard projective techniques on 10th April, 1951. These techniques were the Rorschach, the Thematic Apperception Test and the Rotter Incomplete Sentences.

Rorschach

Mrs. J.'s Rorschach performance suggests that she has above average intellectual ability (approximately 125 I.Q.). Her intelligence is primarily of a 'sponge-like' nature; not particularly original nor creative. She tends toward slight over-generalization, toward the solution of problems by 'principles' rather than flexible situation-by-situation solutions.

Mrs. J.'s perceptual-cognitive rapport with reality is excellent. She tends to perceive things similarly to other persons in her culture without being slavishly conforming.

In spite of a superior over-all adjustment, she tends to be somewhat anxious and sensitive. One would expect an excellent social façade covering slight feelings of inadequacy. She would probably be characterized in her interpersonal relationships as competent and adequate though slightly reserved. She would not be expected to be especially hostile. Her hostility would tend to be expressed obliquely rather than openly. While she is somewhat emotional, her emotions are well controlled. And while slightly shy and sensitive, she tends to be externally, rather than internally, oriented.

According to two sign approach scoring systems of adjustment, Mrs. J.'s protocol is above average when compared with the total group of the mothers in this study. She had only one of Harrower-Erickson's 'neurotic signs', fewer than the mean of the mothers in this study. Mrs. J. had ten of Davidson's 'signs of adjustment', considerably more than the average mother in this study.

Thematic Apperception Test

(i) Daughter role: Mrs. J.'s stories suggest that she was closer to her mother than her father. The father was described as benign and innocuous. Her mother was seen as emotionally supporting but dominating. Mrs. J. seemed to have considerable ambivalence towards her mother, especially concerning independence-dependence. The mother and daughter seem to have been mutually supporting in certain situations. One would expect considerable difficulty on Mrs. J.'s part in attempting to break with her mother at the time of the marriage. The break was probably relatively decisive overtly but there seem to be lingering dependent ties, some of which are not too acceptable to Mrs. J. She still, however, is looking to both parents for recognition in her role as wife and mother.

(ii) Mother role: Mrs. J.'s stories suggest that she attempts, and succeeds, in being less dominating toward her children than her own mother was toward her. This does not seem to be through emotional over-reaction but rather through an intellectualized series of generalizations of what is good for the children. This is accomplished without either the extreme of rigid, authoritarian 'rule setting' or of 'grit your teeth and bear it' intellectualized permissiveness. She tends to be slightly lacking in natural warmth and understanding of the children but, on the whole, has established a comfortable relationship in which she tends to give considerable instrumental aid; less direct emotional support. Generally she feels competent in, and derives considerable satisfaction from, her mother and housewife roles. She is neither excessively anxious and over-protective nor excessively rejecting. What little overt hostility she directs toward her children tends to be mild and oblique and relatively free from feelings of guilt.

(iii) Wife role: There are slight indications of some anxiety and hostility toward men. While this seems to be pervasive, it is extremely mild. Her stories suggest that she takes a slightly nurturant role toward her husband who is seen as relatively less competent than herself. The marital relationship seems to be a very compatible one though somewhat lacking in a free and easy demonstration of affection and closeness.

(iv) Self: On the whole, Mrs. J. sees her environment as friendly and accepting. When the environment is seen as somewhat threatening, she makes a marked effort to minimize the threat. She sees herself as a generally competent person deriving considerable satisfactions in her interpersonal relationships. Her major controlling defence is the utilization of a sometimes conscious attitude of 'things aren't bad, they'll turn out all right'.

Rotter Incomplete Sentences

In this projective technique the subject is asked to complete sentences such as 'I like . . ', 'I regret . . ', 'People . . ', 'Marriage . . . ', etc., 'to express your real feelings'. Using the *Rotter Manual* for college women, Mrs. J. obtained a raw score of 102 (low score suggesting adjustment, with the median score for mothers in this study being 136). Mrs. J.'s score was approximately two standard deviations above the mean of the group.

(i) Her parents: Mrs. J.'s only description of her father is completely positive, 'a wonderful and understanding person'. She again expresses ambivalence toward her mother; contrast 'A mother is one who stands by you', with 'I regret my mother isn't more understanding of young people'.

(ii) Wife and Mother: This is an area of much satisfaction. She has thoroughly accepted these roles as worth while and enjoyable. She sees the family as a closely knit organization of interdependent satisfactions.

(iii) Self: She expresses considerable self-confidence and self-satisfaction. She tends to desire a nurturant role toward close relevant persons in her environment and toward people in general. Not only is there a freedom from conflict, friction and complaint in her sentences, but also, conversely, she gives many statements of positive satisfactions in diverse areas of her life. She is quite sensitive, especially toward persons whom she considers lacking in consideration. While this hypersensitivity seems to be pervasive (and possibly a reason for her inability to be openly warm and accepting), it leads to no perceptions of major environmental threats. Again there is evidence of an intellectualized minimization of threat; again with no strong effort or tension going into this control mechanism.

(d) Pre-Natal Nutrition

Child's Name—Bruce, J. Delivery Date, 3rd June, 1943.

Dietary Supplements:

    1st April, through ninth month, Halibut liver oil, 1 capsule daily.

Pre-pregnancy Weight: 57·61 kg.

         Height: 168.9 cm.

Total Weight Gain: 7·24 kg.

No. of complete weeks diet records kept: 16

Reliability: Good. Detailed records, occasionally amounts not specific.

AVERAGE DAILY DIETARY INTAKE

		Pregnancy 1–27 weeks	requirements 28–40 weeks	Approx. range[1] within this study	Mrs. J.
Calories		2,300	2,600	1,650–2,800	2,334
Protein (gm)		70	80	55–85	82
Minerals					
Ca	(gm)	0·7	1·4	0·6–1·2	0·8
P	(gm)	1·3	1·6	1·0–1·6	1·4
Fe	(mg)	20	20	11·0–16·4	18·0
Vitamins					
A	(IU)	4,000	9,000	4,700–8,900	6,847
B₁	(IU)	200	400	300–450	484
C	(mg)	20	75	65–140	134
D	(IU)	300	800	30–80	67
G	(SB)	500	1,000	500–930	736

[1]Within 1 Standard Deviation.

SUMMARY:

Mrs. J. is an attractive, healthy-looking young woman. She had 'kidney trouble' and constipation early in this pregnancy. Her diet was generous, interesting, and varied. It was low in milk, 5·5 servings per week, and egg, 1·5, and high in sweets, 24·4, and meat, 11·6, and ample in other essential foods.

SIGMA INDEX

(e) Abstracts from Medical Records

FOETAL BEHAVIOUR

Bruce, J. Birth Date, 3rd June, 1943

STANDARD SCORES—MAY 1944 NORMS

Measure	Average last 2 months	1st month before	2nd month before
Heart Rate	50	49	49
Foetal Activity			
1. Total	53	64	44
2. Rhythmic	52	45	49
3. Quick	64	78	50
4. Slow	46	47	43
Mothers Weekly Summary			
1. Too little sleep			
2. Listless, no pep			
3. High spirits on waking			
4. Physically active			
5. Socially active			
6. High strung, tense			
7. Foetus seldom active			
8. Foetus violent			
9. Blue, depressed			
10. Not easily tired			
11. Seldom desire to cry			
12. Fall asleep easily			
13. Much dreaming			

INTERPRETATION

The activity of the foetus, in terms of the norms used, was approximately average during the eighth month of pregnancy. However, during the ninth month the foetal activity, in terms of quickness, reached a standard score of 78 or 2·8 standard deviations above the mean. No other values deviated significantly from the mean.

(f) *Pre-Natal and Labour Summary*

PRE-NATAL SUMMARY:

This was Mrs. J.'s fourth pregnancy, the second full-term pregnancy. The first and third pregnancies were miscarriages, the second pregnancy ended in a still-birth. She had constipation and urinary disturbances throughout this pregnancy. There were no other complaints. She was emotionally happy throughout the pregnancy.

SUMMARY OF LABOUR RECORD:

Child born: 12.20 a.m. Date: 3rd June, 1943.

Length of labour: $3\frac{1}{2}$ hours.

Presentation and position: Occiput left anterior.

Method of delivery: Low forceps apparently used. Episiotomy.

Medication before delivery: Demerol 100 mg.; scopolamine gs. 1/150.

Post-partum medication: Ergotrate 1 cc.

Anaesthetic: Nitrous Oxide and ethylene.

Respiration: No difficulties in establishing respiration.

Condition of infant: Good.

Birth-weight: 8.7 lb.

(g) *Parent Behaviour rating*

Name: Bruce J. Date rated: 21st November, 1945. Age in months: 29

Variable	Sigma Index	Low 20	30	40	Average 50	60	High 70	80	
Adjustment of home:	Maladjusted					• -			Well-adjusted
Activeness of home:	Inactive				•				Active
Discord in home:	Harmony			•		.			Conflict
Sociability of family:	Reclusive		•						Expansive
Co-ordination of household:	Chaotic				•				Co-ordinated
Child-centredness of home:	Child-subordinated				•				Child-centred
Duration of contact with mother:	Brief contact					•			Extensive contact
Intensity of contact with mother:	Inert					• -			Vigorous
Restrictiveness of regulations:	Freedom					• -			Restriction
Readiness of enforcement:	Lax			•					Vigilant

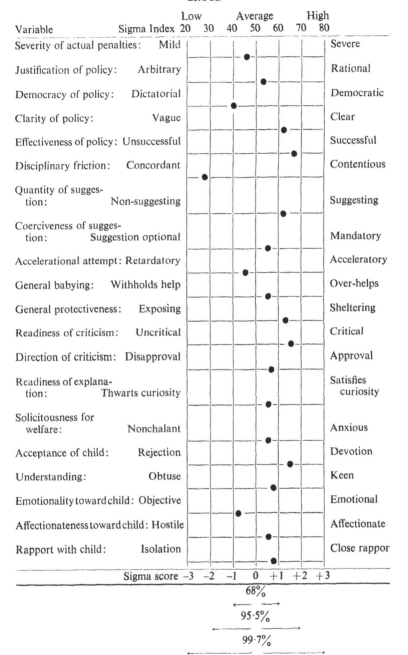

Variable	Sigma Index	Low 20 30	Average 40 50 60	High 70 80	
Severity of actual penalties:	Mild				Severe
Justification of policy:	Arbitrary				Rational
Democracy of policy:	Dictatorial				Democratic
Clarity of policy:	Vague				Clear
Effectiveness of policy:	Unsuccessful				Successful
Disciplinary friction:	Concordant				Contentious
Quantity of suggestion:	Non-suggesting				Suggesting
Coerciveness of suggestion:	Suggestion optional				Mandatory
Accelerational attempt:	Retardatory				Acceleratory
General babying:	Withholds help				Over-helps
General protectiveness:	Exposing				Sheltering
Readiness of criticism:	Uncritical				Critical
Direction of criticism:	Disapproval				Approval
Readiness of explanation:	Thwarts curiosity				Satisfies curiosity
Solicitousness for welfare:	Nonchalant				Anxious
Acceptance of child:	Rejection				Devotion
Understanding:	Obtuse				Keen
Emotionality toward child:	Objective				Emotional
Affectionateness toward child:	Hostile				Affectionate
Rapport with child:	Isolation				Close rappor

Sigma score −3 −2 −1 0 +1 +2 +3

68%

95·5%

99·7%

RECORDS OF BRUCE HIMSELF

(a) *Home Visits*

1st Home Visit—20th October, 1943. 9–11 a.m.

Bruce, age 4 months.

This was the first home visit made to the J.s. Bruce is their first living child though Mrs. J. has had two miscarriages previously and one still-birth. The doctor who took care of her for these pregnancies and deliveries also delivered Bruce. No reason was discovered for her past difficulties in carrying the babies to term or for the one that was born dead. The doctor has recommended that she go ahead and have another baby right away, now that she has had a successful pregnancy and birth. She is uncertain as to the feasibility of this, partly for financial reasons and partly because she thinks she might not feel well during another pregnancy and would not be as patient as she should be with Bruce.

Bruce's birth-weight was 8 lb 7 oz. He was judged to be a healthy sound baby at first. He was put on a formula almost from the first for reasons for which I neglected to interview. Before Bruce came home from the hospital he began to have trouble keeping his feedings down. A scheme was tried whereby he would receive more feedings but smaller in quantity. Once he was home, Mrs. J. found that she couldn't get him to keep more than two ounces of milk down at a time. Anything more than that he would throw up. She was terribly concerned, 'almost frantic', because a nurse at the hospital had told her that she had been able to give him four ounces at a time. Whenever Bruce did get too much he would vomit it expulsively so that the undigested milk would be coughed up with force. It was a terrifying thing for this mother who had had such difficulties in the past.

During Bruce's second week it was recommended that he return to the hospital for examinations to determine the cause of his difficulty. It was found that the pyloric sphincter was too small, and that an operation would be necessary. A long incision was made on the right side from above the navel extending well below it. The operation was a fairly simple one but took several weeks in the hospital to heal. He was about a month old when he came home from the hospital. At first he was given frequent small feedings preceded by a dose of atropine to relax the muscles of the gastro-intestinal tract. He was kept on atropine until about his third month. When he is particularly upset or particularly tired even now he sometimes vomits his feeding, but it is happening less frequently than before.

At the present time he has four meals a day, sleeping long hours between the feedings, which the doctor says is the best possible thing for him to do. He even is able to forgo the 11 p.m. feeding, and has been able to for over a month. He receives about 7 oz. at a feeding, plus about an ounce which is put in his cereal food, which he likes soupy. He has been receiving strained fruits and vegetables for the past few weeks. He likes them fairly well, but often refuses them. When he does so, Mrs. J. doesn't force him at all, excludes them for several days, and then re-introduces them into his diet.

Mrs. J. said that Bruce is a particularly anxious baby because of his difficult first few months. He tires particularly easily, is upset by deviation from routine, is bothered by noises. Mrs. J. upbraided herself for being over-confident about his hardiness last week when she took him to an afternoon birthday party at the home of her sister-in-law. At first she had qualms about attending the party but was urged to do so by her mother-in-law who lives near by. Bruce was over-stimulated at the party by so much adult attention, and later, when he had been put down for his nap, by the noises made by the other children. He screamed and cried all afternoon, was thoroughly exhausted that evening, could hardly eat his meal.

Also when he was at the clinic at the age of three months, the first and third month visits were combined so that he was put through a particularly fatiguing session. He cried so hard and so long that he couldn't stop sobbing until hours after she got him home. After this session he slept for six hours without waking or demanding food. The doctor has told her to take it particularly easy with him and to see that he leads the most routine of existences, to let him sleep all he needs, never waking him for a meal, never to startle or stimulate him unnecessarily. Mrs. J. is trying to follow these instructions as closely as she can. For example, this morning when she bathed him she explained that she doesn't really put him into the water, but rather, just gives him a sponge-bath because he seemed to be startled by the amount of lack of support that being put into water represented.

I was surprised to hear Mrs. J. say that in spite of the difficulties she had with past pregnancies she assumed all through this latest one that everything would be all right. Her attitude during and shortly after Bruce's operation was similarly optimistic. She never doubted but that he'd be all right. She is a particularly happy-seeming person, serene, and secure. She was holding Bruce in her arms when I arrived, saying that he has been off schedule since the birthday party and that I was lucky this morning because he woke up late so hadn't had his bath or bottle. He is on a strictly self-demand schedule. His bath equipment is upstairs, so we went there to start the bath. Mrs. J. said that she loves to care for him, and showed it in the way she treated him throughout the performance of his routine. She *really* wanted this baby. After the bath, which he submitted to, but did not particularly enjoy, he had his meal.

Mrs. J. held him in her arms to give him his milk and cereal. She pointed out the fact to me that he was making an attempt to hold the bottle himself. He has been doing this for about a month. He seems to like, too, to help guide the spoon containing cereal to his mouth. This, too, is permitted though it considerably slows the feeding process and is very messy. Mrs. J. is deft, sure, relaxed, and happy as she takes care of him. After he was fed she put him to bed upstairs in a 'snuggle ducky'.[1] He fell asleep immediately.

This seems like a particularly happy home. Mrs. J. spoke of some of the pleasant activities that she and her husband enjoy. They have a wide circle of friends whom they see frequently at week-ends. Mrs. J.'s family home is in a nearby city where she still has friends and relations whom she sees regularly. Their home is an attractive one, rather small but very pleasant. It is a double house. They have a living-room, dining-room, and kitchen downstairs, and two bedrooms and a bath upstairs. Six months out of the year Mrs. J.'s mother lives with them and six months she lives with a sister of Mrs. J.'s. She is not with them at this time nor will she be this winter.

2nd Home visit—3rd January, 1944. 9–11 a.m.

Bruce, age 7 months.

Bruce has recovered 100 per cent from his early difficulties. In every respect he is a healthy normal child. He is particularly attractive, plump, responsive, bright-eyed. At the time of the former home visit, Mrs. J. had to be very careful that he got an over-abundance of rest and quiet. She had to keep him away from over-stimulating situations. Now she can take him with her to the parties that she and her husband attend and be sure that he will not be too tired when they are over. She is still cautious about introducing him to strange and unknown events, of course, but probably would have been, anyway. She often leaves him with her mother or with one of his aunts when she has plans which cannot include him. He shows little fear of strangers.

At seven months he has four teeth, two having erupted on his six-month birthday, the other two at seven months. He is strong, able to stand in his 'teeter-babe',[2] rolls over, etc. He first rolled over from back to stomach in October at four months. His mother has carefully noted in his baby-book each event in his life.

[1] An envelope, made of blanket material, into which the baby is placed.
[2] A little chair with a canvas seat attached to a very flexible metal frame.

It is quite obvious that Mrs. J. is very happy taking care of him. She bathed him this morning while I was there. Both she and Bruce enjoyed the situation tremendously. He has no fear of the water because she introduced him to tub-baths very gradually. She started out giving him nothing but sponge-baths. She then promoted him to the sling that fits in the bathinette. By now he is enjoying sitting in the bathinette, being splashed, doesn't even seem alarmed when he slips and gets his ears or the back of his head in the water.

Bruce is supposed to be on three meals a day. Mrs. J., however, does give him an extra bottle about 4 p.m. She had trouble getting him to take any vegetables. She tried them in increasing quantity with his cereal, which he loves, which seemed to work well. She still has to dilute the strong flavour of the strained baby vegetables with cereal. He eats fairly readily, weighs as much as he should. His schedule is a particularly regular and predictable one. He wakens at 6.30 or so in the morning, has his breakfast, returns to bed until 9. In the evening he plays for half an hour or so, gets his bath, goes back to bed about 7. He always sleeps on his back, has done so since he was born. If on his stomach, he cries until turned, or rolls over by himself. The fact that he turns his head from side to side while sleeping has kept his head in good shape. He has been sleeping with a toy rabbit which was given to him as an Easter gift by his grandmother. He had it in bed with him this morning. He holds one of its soft ears against his cheek, puts his thumb in his mouth and falls asleep readily. He seems to demand having the little soft toy every time he is put down to sleep. He sometimes takes a little nap in his play-pen in the middle of the day.

Thus far, then, the parents of Bruce are wholly approving and satisfied with their son's development and personality. Their whole life centres around him, though they don't deny themselves sociability on his account. Mrs. J. recently purchased an expensive set of *The Book of Knowledge*[1] for Bruce's use as he grows older. Her husband was horrified and a little disapproving of the price she had to pay for it. However, she wants him to have every advantage and every facility that he might want or need. Mrs. J. reports that Bruce is almost the tallest of his three cousins that were born so close together. He is the youngest of the three but has developed physically at a faster rate than the other two. He was also very tall at birth. She had some disapproving comments to make about the manner in which one of the children is being handled. She says that the child is afraid of strangers, makes a terrible fuss whenever anyone else takes care of her. She is especially afraid of men. Mrs. J. is glad that Bruce is willing to accept other people.

[1] An encyclopaedia for children.

3rd Home Visit—14*th April*, 1944.

Bruce, age 10 *months.*

After all the initial difficulties with Bruce's feeding he is now getting along fine. There is no trouble with food or anything else, Mrs. J. was confident. Bruce certainly looks healthy, has a firm build, clear skin, pink cheeks and sparkling eyes.

He is still getting his milk from a bottle. Their doctor told Mrs. J. to start weaning him at nine months, but she kept him on the bottle until after his vaccination in case he had trouble with that. He is eating chopped foods and those from the family table that he can manage. He is very hungry for breakfast but won't eat other meals if he is watched, other people being too engrossing. Mrs. J. gave him some milk from the bottle before she put him down for his nap. She pointed out to me how he puts his thumb in his mouth to hold the nipple and drinks that way. She sat down holding him to give him some water, but assured me that she does not rock him to sleep. He cried a bit when she put him in the bed; she tucked him in and left him and he stopped shortly after we got downstairs again. Earlier she had told me how well Bruce sleeps through the night. When it was mentioned that his cousin awakens frequently during the night, Mrs. J. told me that the doctor had told her sister (the child's mother) that rocking her to sleep was not good and that she woke up for more attention. Also she does not wake up when her father puts her to bed. Mrs. J. did not criticize her sister at all, but said she did not believe in 'too much handling' and thinks she is doing the right thing.

Bruce can stand well holding on to low furniture, wavers when he has no support. He finally got the idea when Mrs. J. tried to teach him that he could stoop to pick up things. Now he will squat to get objects on the floor. When he is sitting he will pivot to reach a desired object but will not crawl after it if it rolls out of reach; he has never crawled much, seems fairly cautious. Mrs. J. spoke observantly of the different kinds of walking and crawling friends' children had done, but was not eager to accelerate Bruce. He has appropriate and attractive toys which are kept in a shoe-box which he likes particularly to fit together and push around. Mrs. J. said he can play by himself, and though she is with him much of the time, thinks it is a good thing that he does not have to be 'amused' constantly. She enriches his play without being overpoweringly suggestive, keeps specified things for him, not letting him make just anything a toy whether it is suitable or not. An attractive child, he smiled much, was responsive to his mother, and did much babbling. His exploration did not take him away from one spot but he was visually sensitive, interested in seeing both a person and her image in the mirror at the same time.

Mrs. J. has read quite a bit on child care. She spoke of not having done much outside the home since Bruce's advent. This is because she enjoys so much caring for him and feels that it won't be long before he goes off to school and she won't be able to see so much of him. As she deftly administered the routine she told me how she 'loves bath time'. She was warm but did not shower much overt attention on him while I was there.

She has intellectualized her theories and ideas about child raising. Since Bruce is such a coveted child, the J.s having had so much trouble having a child at all, she realizes the danger of his being 'spoiled' and is particularly anxious to avoid this. She appears thoroughly confident in her own abilities and eager to keep the control of him largely in her own hands. As to grandparents, she frankly said she thought 'each generation has a right to raise its own'. Her mother-in-law, who had arrived the day before to spend the summer with them, seemed to be in accord with this view. A meek and shy little person, she contributed rarely to the conversation, explained to me that she cannot handle or care for the baby because her hands are badly crippled with arthritis. She does do crocheting. She seemed to be an unobtrusive person, but her daughter-in-law, while not resentful of her presence, did not particularly include her in the family circle.

Nor does Mrs. J. consider that the father should have any care of his young son. This I think was more a concept of roles than a selfish attitude. As he has little time when he can be with Bruce he has handled him rarely and does not even know how to dress or undress him. He put him to sleep with all his clothes on, on one rare occasion when she left the child with him. The father enjoys him now that he is big enough to play with, but felt awkward during the infant period. He is *their* child, but his care is *her* job.

Mrs. J. is an entirely pleasant person and satisfied. She spoke of her earlier pregnancies with no morbidity, said she felt the best she ever had during pregnancy. She has not retained her rural point of view or colloquialisms of speech, is quite urbanized, much more socially conversational than her sisters. When knitting was mentioned and I asked if she did any, she replied, not any more. She spends what recreational time she has, reading, thinking it more worth while.

Most of her social associations are connected with their church group, and she takes part in various activities there. She is a somewhat meticulous housekeeper and mother without being fussy. She rarely has others care for Bruce, nor would she travel with him. One time she left him with a neighbour when they went away for a weekend, but they took no vacation. About his first outing, other than to a family gathering, was a recent dinner at a restaurant, which he enjoyed.

4th Home Visit—30th August, 1944. 9.15–11.30 a.m.

  Bruce, age 14 *months.*

Bruce came up to see what was happening as his mother opened the door for me and took my coat. As soon as we took notice of him and talked to him, however, he became self-conscious and shy. For the remainder of the morning he was apprehensive about me, though cheerful. Mrs. J. said that he always needs to take his time to warm up to people and that he is really disturbed if they swoop down upon him, a usual thing at his age. He is socially oriented, more interested in taking things to show to his mother and grandmother and having some sort of contact with them, than in playing with the materials that he has. He looked me all over too. He has a few words that are almost distinguishable now: 'Hello' and 'How do?'

Bruce has been walking since he was eleven months but he has never crawled. When he is seated or falls down he cannot get up by himself. Mrs. J. always helps him, and the reason that she thinks he wouldn't pull himself up at all, no matter how long she left him, is that he does not get up even in his crib where he has the sides to hold on to. People have told her that if she let him struggle for himself he would learn. She is a little concerned that he has not developed more rapidly in this line but does feel that he is all right. He is always happy when she finds him lying in his crib, is not particularly frustrated by his inability to get up by himself.

Some of the toys he has do not appeal to him at all yet. The thing Bruce enjoys most is to get out some of the kitchen pots, pans and spoons. Mrs. J. has designed one cupboard that he can explore, keeps the others tied so that he cannot get into them. Mrs. J. was ironing while I was there, but was willing to interrupt her work at any time to look at things that Bruce brought her or to show him a picture book. He has several very nice picture books, and Mrs. J. says that they always look at one together before she puts him in bed: this applies to nap time as well as at night. She goes through and points out specific items in the pictures, and he recognizes these in his favourite books that he has seen most often. Mrs. J. says that she does not take him outside at all to play in the wintertime.

Bruce has his bath in the big tub now, thoroughly enjoying it, bobbing bath-toys in the water but without any vigorous splashing. Mrs. J. seems to enjoy this process, still going through the complete routine of oiling him all over, etc. The mother is able to put considerable effort into cleanliness, without over-emphasizing its importance. Bruce had never had a cold, except for slight sniffles, until just before his first birthday. The big celebration of his birthday at his grand-mother's was very exciting for him. All the other grandchildren were there, and they tried to take movies of them all and Bruce was pretty well worn out by the end of it.

Mrs. J. tried weaning Bruce at nine months but gave it up as un-successful. Then on 3rd June (she remembered the exact date!), she tried it again and accomplished the change-over to a cup almost over-night. She quotes her doctor on all measures, seems to have great faith in him and to follow instructions quite implicitly. Bruce does a small amount of thumb-sucking. When I asked about feeding, Mrs. J. said that everything is going fine, but with more details it proved not to be so simple. She is not worried or bothered by the extra fuss. Bruce does not take any fruits very well except apple. Spinach and carrots she usually mixes with cereal and milk or potato so that he will eat them more readily. Meat she cuts very fine, and tries to stick mainly to things that she knows are more easily digested. She lets him feed himself, especially if it is a food that he does not especially care for.

Mrs. J. puts him on a potty for bowel movements, since he has them quite regularly after meals, two or sometimes three, times a day. She has used a suppository when he has not defecated for a day or so. She has started no training for urination, plans to wait until he is fifteen or sixteen months old. Here again she quoted her doctor as authority, but was much in accord with the theory of not starting too early. She has plenty of confidence in her own ability but is backed up by the doctor's views too.

Mrs. J. is going into a local hospital at the end of the month for an operation for haemorrhoids. She has had trouble with this for some time and is relieved to feel that it is going to be taken care of. Bruce will stay with his grandmother, and his father will probably sleep there too. That is the arrangement that will be easiest for Bruce since he likes his grandmother and easily warms up to her, whereas it takes him much longer with anyone else even though he sees them quite frequently. When I suggested something about Bruce's missing her, Mrs. J. said that she'd probably miss him more than he would her. She is very affectionate, cherishes him as a quite precious possession.

Mr. J.'s mother, who is now staying with them, will go to another son's while her daughter-in-law is in the hospital. A very quiet and feeble person, she seems to be welcome in the home but is not con-sidered at all in decisions. There seems to be no closeness between the two women, even little conversation, but also no contention at all. She did not come out of the kitchen where she was sitting until her daughter-in-law asked her if she would like to join us in the living-room, and then she was hardly included in what was said. While I was there Mr. J.'s brother's wife called and Mrs. J. told her of the operation and asked if it would be all right to have the elder Mrs. J. stay with her. After the call Mr. J.'s mother was told what had been decided, as if she had not been consulted at all before, or even told what they expected to do. The relationship between the mother-in-law and daughter-in-law appears odd as it is marked by such complete passivity, while they are living so closely together. Any regard or resentment that might be felt is entirely covered by neutrality, I noticed both on this and my prior visit with them.

5th Home Visit—21st November, 1945.

Bruce, age 29 months.

Change in home: David born, 3rd October, 1945.

According to Mrs. J. everything has gone well with David's development. They have had no difficulty getting him established on a formula and he has gained steadily. The mother started nursing him, but did not have enough milk to satisfy him. He did not care about having any breast-milk when supplementary feedings were added, Mrs. J. said, so he was switched over to the bottle entirely. Mrs. J. considers him a greedy eater. She followed her doctor's directions explicitly in preparing the formula, just two days ago increased the proportion of milk to water. It consists of canned evaporated milk, corn syrup and water. David had spit up his first bottle this morning and Mrs. J. thought it must be because she had made a mistake in measuring the ingredients for the formula and got it too rich. He has spit up before but she does not consider it anything to get alarmed about.

David takes about 7½ oz. from four bottles a day and 5 oz. from the last one in the evening. He had his first bottle at 4.30 this morning, then the second one was not until 10. He usually sleeps from 8.30 or 9 p.m. until the early morning feeding. Mrs. J. declared that she sometimes feels guilty about how little she picks David up and holds him. He rarely cries and needs little attention to see that he is cared for. She fed him in a leisurely way today, talked to him approvingly and cuddled him. He was awake all the time that I was there, just beginning to doze off about the time I was leaving, which was at least a half-hour after he'd finished his bottle. He seemed to be a content and aware infant though not highly active.

Bruce was told before the advent that a new sib was arriving. Mrs. J. did not think it meant much to him and says that he is interested in the baby now. During the time that I was there Bruce ignored his brother except when Mrs. J. suggested that he look at him or pat him before she took him off to bed for his nap. She keeps most of David's equipment downstairs except for the bed in which he sleeps, so that Bruce is apt to be around while David is being fed or cared for. Since one of his cousins was there for the morning, Bruce was playing with him. Ordinarily Bruce may take more notice of the baby. He stayed at his maternal grandmother's while Mrs. J. was in the hospital, and Mrs. J. hired a woman to help her for about the first three weeks after she came home from the hospital. Since he sees quite a bit of his grandparents it was not a great change for him to be with them, except that it was for a more prolonged time. Mrs. J. thought there was no evidence of his really missing her, though she missed him. The only change she noted was that when she and the baby were first home Bruce had toilet accidents more often than usual. But that is now back to the previous state of a few rare daytime and night accidents.

Mrs. J. says that she feels very well now, and does not feel that the delivery was very hard on her. She contrasted her own real missing of Bruce this time to her session in the hospital September a year ago for a haemorrhoid operation, when she did not even think about him. That was so painful for about three weeks, she said, that she did not care whether she lived or died. She thinks it disgraceful now that she thought so little about home.

The cousin was there for the morning and Mrs. J. supervised their play closely, being highly suggestive as to what they should do to keep the play materials divided evenly and used in such a way as not to mar furniture. She described Bruce as 'good natured' and submissive. The cousin was more dominant, took the toys he wanted and was more apt to reject Mrs. J.'s suggestions. She was conscientious about seeing that neither one took something the other was using first, and when there was a conflict over a tractor and she did not know who had had it first, she took it away and gave them both other toys.

The play was very peaceful with neither one getting excited or demanding. Whenever Bruce wanted an object that wasn't currently available, he asked Mrs. J. for it. He is quiet-mannered, yet not passive, laughed readily but did no whimpering, readily accepted his mother's suggestions when he understood them. She considers that, with the two of them, she has to be especially watchful to keep two steps ahead of them to prevent anything dangerous or destructive. Bruce frequently plays outside now, often asking to go out as soon as he awakens.

There is a five-year-old child who lives across the street who sometimes plays with Bruce. Mrs. J. considers her very spoiled and selfish, said she does not like him to associate with her too much, but thinks he will have to be able to get along with all types of children. The child calls to him to come over, and he is too young for the explanation that there are times when he can and can't go. Bruce's vocabulary sounded about usual for a two-and-a-half-year-old and his words were fairly distinct, though there were a few that Mrs. J. did not understand. The mother is interested in his intellectual development, said she had difficulty explaining on his level the things he is beginning to ask about, e.g. where is the moon in the daytime and what are clouds?

(b) Observations during September 1947 Nursery School Visits

Bruce was breast-fed for one week after birth: within that time, he became a feeding-problem, vomiting and spitting up all milk. A formula was substituted for breast-feeding, as it was thought the breast milk was causing the disturbance; but shortly thereafter the infant was found to have a pyloric stenosis. An operation was performed, and atropine was administered for two months until the vomiting disappeared. Within a short time after the operation, the infant was reported as having a good appetite, although he still vomited his feedings when particularly upset or tired. On the advice of her physician, Mrs. J. gave Bruce frequent but small feedings, with long hours of sleep between each feeding.

Strained foods and vegetables were introduced into the diet at about three and a half months.

At three months, the mother reported that the child was attempting to hold his bottle, and to help guide the spoon to his mouth for feedings. She encouraged him in this.

Weaning from the bottle was begun at ten months, and the changeover to a cup was almost immediate, although a small amount of thumb-sucking still continued.

Bruce has shown no food allergies. He dislikes all fruits except apple. His appetite is now reported as good.

Toilet-training for bowel movements was begun at nine months. Training for urination was begun at eighteen and completed at twenty-two months.

For a short time after the advent of the new baby (David), Bruce (twenty-nine months) had more toilet accidents, but this soon cleared up.

Mrs. J. uses a suppository when Bruce has not defecated for a day or so.

(c) Feeding Behaviour and Toilet-Training

Bruce, age 36 *months.*

Nursery Play Observations

The nursery group:

Age range of group of nine children was from 36 to 42 months; Bruce was the youngest.

Bruce's group status and play with group members:

Bruce related almost constantly to Jimmy (a child he knew before coming to nursery school). Much associative and co-operative play with Jimmy (thirty-three of forty-six observation periods of three minutes each). During several other periods, he watched Jimmy a lot or tried to join play with him, with Jimmy ignoring or rejecting. Considerable play also with Barbara A. and Bobby N.

Bruce was not generally very well liked in the group. He was often interfering or aggressive in his approaches to others. He was quite often ignored or rejected, although other children did often follow him to play with him. During the third week of nursery school, Jimmy more often ignored or rejected him than accepted him.

Bruce's types of play:

He played alone less than the average for the group (rank 7— rank 1 is high). He had a high degree of associative and co-operative play, chiefly with Jimmy (rank 1 in group). He sought to join others in play often (rank 1 in overtures to other children).

Vigour of Bruce's play:

His play was highly vigorous with much running and yelling. He was always on the go. He ranked third in vigour among all thirty-six nursery children in the four age groups (rank 1 in his group).

Dependency devices:

He showed a strong orientation toward children rather than teachers as far as dependent responses were concerned. Only 19 per cent. of his dependent responses were directed toward adults in the nursery. His orientation toward children is shown by his ranks in the dependent categories given below:

	Teacher	Child
Clinging, hanging around . . .	8	3
Seeking attention	7	3
Seeking approval	8	2
Seeking acceptance (total of above)	8	1
Imitating other children . . .		1

In just one area did Bruce show equal teacher-child orientation—noticing stimuli from teachers and children elsewhere in the nursery. He ranked highest in the group both in watching teachers and watching other children.

Independence behaviour :

In self-reliance: as measured by intensity of alone-play, Bruce ranked lowest in the group. He was highly distractible and lacked persistence, rarely staying with an activity for as long as one minute.

In self-assertion: Bruce had a high rating (rank 1 in the group) in attempts to direct other children. These attempts were often ignored or rejected. He was about average in interfering with others' play or in aggression. He resisted interference or aggression by others less frequently than the average (rank 6 in the group).

Defences:

It is difficult to identify Bruce's reactions to rejected dependence. If one considers his reactions when his overtures to others were ignored or rejected, the answer is that he was often persistent, repeating the overture; frequently ingratiating (bringing a toy, etc.); very often attention-seeking by loud play, etc. Frequently, on rejection, he turned toward another child, seeking to join play with him. On one occasion, he attacked the child whom Jimmy elected to play with in preference to himself. On a few occasions he interfered with or was aggressive with other children after Jimmy refused to play with him.

Evidence of adjustment level:

Bruce was highly nervous and restless. He was always seeking to establish and maintain play relations with other children. His almost constant watching what went on in the room suggests a lack of security and anxiety about his relations with others. He seemed always under strain to be noticed and accepted. He did little finger-sucking (rank 8 in the group). He smiled a lot (rank 1). Much of the time his smiling and laughing were apparently ingratiation or attention-seeking.

Trip Observations:

Bruce seemed well-adjusted leaving home and driving to the nursery school. He smiled and waved good-bye to his mother on the first day of nursery school. He was rather quiet in the car the first day but smiled and giggled with the others the second day.

Experimental Sessions (15-minute session alone with experimenter):

In performing games and puzzles, Bruce was hesitant and timid about getting started. He asked considerable help, much of it un-

68

necessary or without sufficient trying first. He showed definite physical apprehension walking along a springy board and entering a darkened room alone to get candy. He lacked persistence and flexibility in working with the frustration tasks. Generally, he seemed uncertain and hesitant in his relations with adults, though he maintained contact by a constant stream of conversation.

(d) Behaviour during physical growth examination

The examination consisted of measurements, X-rays, photographs, and a medical examination. Throughout, Bruce was observed and rated by two independent observers. Their rating cards are summarized here.

(i) At 44 months (28th February, 1946)

The observers noted that Bruce cried and called for his mother both as he entered and during the examination. Also that he 'accepted reassurance'. The points on which he was observed and his ratings are as follows:

Physical resistance to manipulation: 'mild', several 'occasional mild' and 'passive'.

Fear or anxiety: one observer rated his behaviour during X-ray as 'terrified', otherwise he seemed 'fearful', with the comment, 'crying, trembled at first, became quieter'.

Anger or resentment: one observer saw him as 'unfriendly' and 'complacent'; the other as 'complacent' and 'friendly', during different parts of the examination.

Emotional dependence on adults: 'occasional clinging' throughout, with one 'frequent clinging' entry.

Activity level: 'passive' throughout.

(ii) At 48 months (7th June, 1947)

According to both observers, Bruce still cried, called for mother and home. He accepted reassurance, though one observer remarked, 'Very apprehensive; continually wanted to know what was coming next. Never seemed completely reassured'. The other noted 'Anxiety at each *change* in procedure'. It was noted that he had a fever and sore throat.

Physical resistance to manipulation: 'passive' throughout except for one entry just inside the 'co-operative' column.

Fear or anxiety: generally 'fearful', occasionally 'somewhat anxious'.

Anger or resentment: generally 'complacent', occasionally 'friendly'.

69

Emotional dependence on adults: one observer stressed 'frequent clinging', the other 'occasional clinging'.

Activity level: 'passive' with one 'periodic activity' entry.

(e) *Abstract of Illness History*

(i) To age 12 months:

Nose, throat, sinus: Mild cold twice, no fever, 'sniffles'. Vaporizer prescribed.

Gastro-intestinal system: Pyloric stenosis from birth.

10th July, 1943: vomited once at noon; not projectile.

12th July, 1943: started projectile vomiting after taking 2 oz. Breast-fed one week. Atropine tried but unsuccessful.

13th July, 1943: vomited 1–1½ hours after feeding. Taken to hospital.

16th July, 1943: Surgery. In hospital three days. Bottle-fed. Vomited about half of feedings. Atropine in hospital and at home.

19th August to 15th September, 1943: Atropine gradually decreased in dosage; finally discontinued. Child getting along well. Vomited only once since. Now fed when cries.

Nervous system: sucks thumb when tired or hungry.

Skin: Impetigo (abdominal wall and down to upper thigh), July 1943, for ten to twelve days. Sulfonamide ointment prescribed.

Teeth: One left lower incisor, 22nd December, 1943.

Immunizations: Triple vaccine, injections 6th January, 9th February, 7th March, 1944. Smallpox vaccination, 8th April, 1944.

Operations and accidents: Circumcision 8th June, 1943. Surgery for pyloric stenosis, 16th July, 1943. In hospital for three days. Good recovery apparently.

(ii) To age 18 months:

Nose, throat, sinus: Mild cold, August, 1944.

Ears: Infection (right ear) following cold above. Penicillin prescribed.

Eyes: At the same time as ear infection, 8th August, 1944, right tear duct closed so that tears do not drain off. Mother instructed to massage area.

Gastro-intestinal system: No intestinal upsets. Bowels normal.

Genito-urinary system: Toilet training just started. Seems quite successful.

Nervous system: Sucks thumb and tickles end of nose at bedtime.

Immunizations: Schick test (for scarlet fever)—negative.

Speech and writing: Trying to talk; not progressing as rapidly as some children.

(iii) To age 24 months:

Nose, throat, sinus: Mild sore throat, 13th March, 1945. Doctor seen, no prescription.

Ears: Moderate infection in both ears. Penicillin prescribed, 16th February, 1945.

(iv) To age 30 months:

Nose, throat, sinus: Moderate cold, 9th August to 12th August, 1945. 101° F. temperature one day. One penicillin injection.

Lymphatic system: Cervical glands swollen with cold above.

Immunizations: 17th July, 1945, booster triple vaccine.

4. SANDRA

Three years old

INTRODUCTION

Of the 1,252 infants housed in the Rooming-In Unit[1] between its opening and the close of the time for selection of study patients, approximately half came from families belonging to the professional or professional-in-training class. The records of three families were selected for the Seminar on Mental Health and Infant Development from the predominant socio-economic group of the rooming-in families, and from this group only, in the belief that the differences in the children and parent-child relationship would stand out more strikingly against a similarity of background. The three sets of parents were alike in the following respects: They were white, of early American descent, and Protestant. They were aged between twenty-five and thirty. They were college graduates, and the husbands were post-graduate students. The pregnancies were planned; the parents all felt they could afford a family and that they could count on help either from their families or from some other source of income. The mothers were primiparas and the infants were female, born within a few months of each other under similar hospital conditions. The mothers were private patients. They had requested rooming-in and wanted to nurse. The parents lived under comparable conditions in a community of families with similar academic background.

The mothers had similar obstetrical care from their obstetricians. They all reported to their obstetrician in the third months of pregnancy. They were seen, according to the obstetrician's routine plan, at monthly intervals through the first six months, at bi-monthly intervals during the seventh and eighth months, and weekly during the ninth month. Since the rooming-in records focus principally on relationships and attitudes, they do not contain definite data on diet prescribed or taken prenatally. It may be assumed, however, that the three mothers received similar advice in respect of diet, limitation of weight gain and personal hygiene. Weight gain is usually limited to

[1]Editor's note: The case of Sandra J. was one of three studied at the Seminar, which were drawn from a Rooming-In Research Project—the designation given to a parent-child relationship study within the framework of the flexible schedule method, as opposed to strict routine, of infant care. It acquired its name from the hospital Rooming-In Unit, a four-bed, semi-private room where mothers and new-born babies are housed together.

72

20 lb., but may be varied according to the mother's physique. Mothers are generally advised to abstain from intercourse and tub bathing during the last six weeks of pregnancy.

All three mothers received the usual hospital care during labour and delivery. Small rooms on the maternity wing are set apart for labour. The husband may remain with his wife in the labour room, but may not accompany her to the delivery room. The mother is shown the baby and permitted to hold him as soon as she feels able. The three mothers had to wait varying intervals before getting into the Rooming-In Unit, for lack of immediate availability of beds.

In addition to the similarity of socio-economic background and exposure to similar suggestions about infant care in the hospital, the three mothers were selected on the basis of one major difference in maternal attitude—a difference in degree of flexibility in their child-care practices.

CASE SUMMARY

(a) Pre-Natal Period

Both the parents of Sandra J. came from families of professional people, and at the time of the present pregnancy, were themselves college graduates studying for advanced degrees and working part-time in professional fields. Mrs. J. was the second of three children, having an older brother and a younger sister. Mr. J. was the oldest of four children, with two younger sisters and a younger brother. The family housing and financial condition were described by the mother as 'adequate' for their present needs. They were living in a very small furnished apartment, which would be unsuitable after the baby came, because of its size. The husband was receiving government assistance as an ex-soldier, and they had some additional financial support from their families.

The mother made application for rooming-in two months prior to her expected date of confinement, explaining that she had read about the service in a local newspaper, and that both she and her husband desired this type of accommodation. She gave as her primary reason for wanting rooming-in the fact that she felt strongly in favour of breast-feeding, and believed having the baby in the room with her would facilitate this. From her reading, she had gathered that infants under the usual separate nursery system were not nursed frequently enough to stimulate the mother's milk supply, and for this reason nursing was often unsuccessful. Mrs. J. expressed herself as feeling 'definitely rebellious' against the idea of formula-feeding, adding in a later interview that her mother was coming to assist her when she returned home from the hospital, and would be distressed if she had to make formula. Both Mrs. J. and her husband were breast-fed, Mrs. J. describing her mother as a 'regular fountain' who nursed all her children up to one year. Mrs. J. stated that her belief in breast-feeding was based on the fact that she had read it was better for the baby, and promoted a more intimate relationship between mother and child. She said her husband felt less strongly on the subject than she did, but was pleased that she wished to breast-feed.

In addition to wanting rooming-in because she felt it would be a help to breast-feeding, Mrs. J. described her desire to have the baby with her as 'instinctive'. Her husband also was in favour of the plan, as he did not want to see the baby 'behind glass', as would be the case if the infant were in the separate nursery. Mrs. J.'s mother had had all her children at home, and Mrs. J. approved of rooming-in because it combined the advantages of home and hospital. She felt the restriction on number of visitors was desirable; visitors might excite her and 'disturb the feeding process'.

Mrs. J. expressed herself as in sympathy with the 'flexible schedule' method, and enumerated several ways in which she would rear her children differently from the way she was brought up. She felt she had been too closely dominated and supervised by her mother; consequently, she would not discipline her children as harshly, or imbue them with fears to make them obedient. She also felt she would give her children more freedom in playing with other children of both sexes; she herself had been forbidden to play with boys.

The pregnancy was planned; the J.s had agreed before marriage that they would like to have a 'large' family (about four children). They wished to wait a year after marriage before having the first because of the numerous other adjustments which would be necessary. The baby was expected twenty-six months after the marriage date, which Mrs. J. described as 'almost on the line'. Mrs. J. did not anticipate that the baby would interfere much with their social activities, as both she and her husband liked to stay home and read. She expressed the hope, however, that after the baby came, she would still have time for the reading.

Mrs. J. enjoyed the baby's movements *in utero* because they were reassuring and gave her a strong sense of personal relationship with the child. She felt that the child had a favourite position, and responded when she herself felt excited about something. Her dreams about the baby had centred around the confinement—e.g., that she had to go to the hospital in a hurry, and that the baby was born rapidly and she was conscious throughout. She expressed no sex preference though at times she felt the child was going to be a girl. Names had been chosen for both boy and girl, but not after any member of either family.

Mrs. J.'s family medical history was marked by diabetes, pernicious anæmia and heart disease in the grandmother, and heart disease and high blood pressure in the mother. Her own general health throughout the pregnancy was good, her routine physical examination negative, and X-ray pelvimetry showed that her bony pelvis was adequate. She experienced severe nausea during the first three months, but she had continued to work at her job as an elementary school teacher during the first four months. She had been somewhat concerned because of the nausea, fearing it would affect the baby's health, but had been reassured on this point by her obstetrician. After the nausea had abated, she had felt 'better and better'. She found her pregnancy 'a great satisfaction' and 'no burden at all'. She was extremely interested in the whole process and, because she was 'an object of great interest to herself', had read extensively. Her husband was also interested, and read the same books (Guttmacher, Deutsch, Read). She felt no anxiety about pregnancy, labour and delivery, partly because she was reassured by her reading, and partly because of her mother's easy labours. Her mother's three labours had all been extremely short, the first lasting half an hour, the second (patient) ten minutes, the third half an hour. Her mother 'would never take any anaesthesia'.

(b) *Labour and Delivery*

According to Mrs. J.'s account, her labour began at about 10 p.m., seven days prior to her expected date of confinement. The initial contractions she described as 'little twinges . . . like menstrual cramps'. By 12 a.m., the contractions were occurring every half hour, and she had a slight 'bloody show', which she recognized from her reading. She was not convinced this was labour, because the contractions were mild and irregular, but called her obstetrician. At 3 a.m., the contractions began to get more frequent, and she began to time them. By 4 a.m., they were between five and twelve minutes apart. At 4.30 a.m. the contractions were three to four minutes apart, and she felt like bearing down. At 5 a.m., she called the doctor and took a taxi to the hospital.

The following account of Mrs. J.'s labour and delivery is abstracted from the hospital chart:

5.15   Entered hospital.
5.30   Membranes intact, strong contractions every 3 to 4 minutes; doctor called.
5.45   Examined by doctor; cervix half dilated, thin; vertex 1 finger breadth below spine.
6   Seconal grs. 3 given; small soapsuds enema.

6.45   Cervix fully dilated, taken to delivery room; patient pushing with contractions; membranes visible at outlet.

7.5   Routine inhalation anaesthesia administered.

7.8   Membranes ruptured artificially; vertex on pelvic floor, advanced with each contraction.

7.16   Delivered spontaneously but with episiotomy, an apparently normal female infant; intramuscular pitocin 1 cc.

7.19   Placenta expressed (Schultze), intact; episiotomy repaired; intramuscular ergotrate 1 cc., estimated blood loss 150 cc.

8.20   Patient in private room, baby to nursery; ergotrate course begun; morphia grs. $\frac{1}{8}$; patient's condition good; fundus firm; lochia moderate.

3.30   Transferred to Rooming-In Unit.

Mrs. J.'s subjective evaluation of her experience is as follows. During the period at home before she came to the hospital, she had not felt that the contractions were particularly painful. She had called the doctor shortly after she went into labour, and felt 'mad' at him for minimizing it. In the hospital, she disliked having to wait for the doctor to arrive; when he did arrive, she told him about her mother's rapid labours. Looking back on her labour, she felt she must have been completely relaxed as at no time did she feel as though she 'had put up a battle'. She found the labour painful but very natural and purposeful, as though she were being 'pushed in that direction'. She remembered the nurse commenting that she could see the baby's head just before she was taken to the delivery room. She felt great satisfaction and relief at being able to bear down, again feeling this 'the most natural thing in the world'. She did not want episiotomy and gas, and would have preferred to be conscious at the delivery. The last thing she remembered before being anaesthetized was saying, 'I want to be present', and 'I don't want that', as the mask was placed over her face. She awoke at 7.45, the forty-minute interval seeming 'like twenty years'. She was told she had a nicely proportioned little girl, and felt very peaceful and triumphant. She had thought it might be a girl, and was pleased. She found the baby, who was to be named Sandra, 'not very pretty, but very cute', and thought she looked like her husband. In retrospect, she felt her optimism during pregnancy about labour and delivery was vindicated, but would have preferred not to be anaesthetized.

(c) *Hospital Period*

Mrs. J. was transferred to the Rooming-In Unit on the afternoon of her delivery day, and remained there until her discharge on her eighth day post-partum. She was not allowed up until her fourth pp.

day, when she was permitted to sit in a chair for fifteen minutes in the morning and afternoon; walking was allowed on the fifth pp. day, and she was allowed to be up as much as she wanted from the sixth day on. She was visited daily by her husband, who came during both the afternoon and evening visiting hours. He is reported to have held the baby frequently, and to have shown considerable interest in the Behaviour Day Sheet kept by his wife.

Mrs. J. nursed the baby as she had planned. She requested that the baby should not be given any formula, so only water was used when the infant seemed dissatisfied after breast-feeding. The baby was first put to breast nine hours after delivery, and sucked well; the mother giggled with delight at her success, because she felt it indicated the child was precocious. Sandra was nursed again one hour later, and then went to sleep. Three hours later, she was observed to be sucking in her crib, but refused the breast. With this one exception, she was reported to suck well and vigorously. The mother nursed sitting up with the baby held flat against her, in a position which seemed awkward to observers. The baby seemed unable to nurse well in any other position, but when held thus, would suck vigorously for twenty minutes or longer, then usually fell asleep. Mrs. J.'s milk came in on the third pp. day, and from then on the baby began to gain weight. Mrs. J. was extremely pleased with the baby's spacing of feedings, and, as early as the first pp. day, felt she could tell when the baby was getting hungry by the degree of restlessness she showed in her sleep. The feeding course was as follows:

Day	No. of Breast Feedings	Total Time	cc. of H_2O	Weight (gms)
DD.	4	1' 45"	43	3,380
1 pp.	5	2' 40"	30	3,225
2 pp.	6	4' 5"	90	3,135
3 pp.	8	4' 20"	?	3,150
4 pp.	7	3' 55"	80	3,280
5 pp.	11	4' 45"	60	3,360
6 pp.	7	2' 42"	15	3,260
7 pp.	5	2' 20"	55	3,360
8 pp. Discharged				3,260

The baby was described as vigorous, chubby, pretty, and generally contented. Mrs. J. was described as having a warm, affectionate attitude toward her, and being very alert to her needs. Although the mother was not permitted up until her fourth pp. day, she asked on the first pp. day if she might care for the baby when she wished to. She showed considerable interest in the Behaviour Day Sheet, studying it to determine what feeding interval most satisfied Sandra. She read Spock, and commented that she felt she had a precocious child because, according to Spock, many children do not find their hands for two or three months, while Sandra slept with hers in her mouth. She planned to enrol Sandra in a noted nursery school, and seemed genuinely upset that she could not do this immediately while she was in the hospital. She kept the baby beside her most of the time, sending her to the nursery on two nights when the infant was crying and disturbing the other mothers in the Unit.

Mrs. J.'s mental attitude was described as generally cheerful, though she was fatigued from meeting the baby's needs. She slept soundly at night, and did not object to being roused to feed the baby. During the fifth night, she cried briefly because she hated to see the baby fussy and crying She also was reported to have once expressed concern about the way she bubbled the baby, because she hated to see Sandra hiccough.

Evaluating her rooming-in experience, Mrs. J. summed it up as an 'unqualified, fundamental success'.

(d) Neo-Natal Period

Mrs. J. was checked at home for one month by the rooming-in paediatrician, who made three visits during this time; the case was then turned over to the private paediatrician she had selected. During the first three weeks, Mrs. J.'s mother was visiting, to help in the home. However, although the father and mother were present at the paediatric visits, the grandmother was not, so her influence could only be inferred from the parents' references to her ideas.

The first post-hospital month was one of alternating periods of confusion and relatively good adjustment. It came out during the first home visit that the first three nights at home were extremely upsetting, as the baby cried and fussed almost constantly. Mrs. J. felt this was primarily because Sandra was hungry, as she herself was fatigued and excited and her milk supply decreased. However, the baby could be given neither formula nor water, since the mother had bought no bottles. Mrs. J. had started to give the baby orange juice the first day at home, but had stopped this because she wondered if it contributed to the baby's fretfulness. The paediatrician advised the mother to resume giving orange juice and to give it during one of the fussy periods between feedings, to offer the baby water, and to take her out during the day. He felt that the baby's self-demand feeding disrupted the family routine, and that the tension was increased by the fact that the grandmother disapproved of such irregularity.

After this initial period, the baby became more regular, and the wakeful nights less frequent. By her twelfth day, the baby was eating every three to four hours, nursing on one breast for twenty to thirty minutes. There followed a period of four to five fussy nights, which again caused the mother concern as to whether she had enough milk. She was reassured by the paediatrician at his second visit that, since the baby was on seven feedings a day, sleeping well between feedings, and gaining weight, all indications were that she was getting enough to eat. The mother was again advised to resume orange juice and to take the baby out during the day, which she had not done. Mrs. J. had begun offering water if the baby seemed dissatisfied after feeds, and was advised by the paediatrician to offer formula occasionally at night so that she could get more rest. Formula was offered for the first time on the baby's twenty-fourth day; the baby took 3 oz. and slept seven hours; this convinced the mother that formula feeding was better than breast-feeding. She still considered the use of supplementary formula inadvisable, but was preoccupied with the thought that she did not have enough milk, and continued to offer the baby one bottle every day, usually in the evening. From this time on, the baby ate five to six times a day (every three to four hours), and frequently slept six hours per night. Mrs. J. was now nursing for twenty minutes on each breast at each feeding.

At the time of the third visit, the mother was again advised to give orange juice between feedings rather than after nursing, which she was doing, and to take the baby out more frequently. The chief topic of conversation at this visit was the mother's concern as to whether she had enough milk, and she was reassured that fluctuations in her supply were to be expected.

Throughout this period, the baby's general health was good. During the first few days at home, she had developed a rash and loose stools, but the rash soon disappeared and the stools became normal. She continued to have a wakeful period in the evening, from 6 p.m. to 10 p.m., during which time the parents played with her.

During the period of his visits, the paediatrician felt that there was considerable friction between the grandmother and the parents, and between husband and wife, over almost all points of the baby's care. Mr. J. was very interested in the baby: as Mrs. J. put it 'a little too interested to suit me'. At each visit, the mother repeated questions about spoiling the baby, feeding, airing, and dressing, and it was apparent that the parents held different views on all these points. In particular, the father asked the paediatrician to assure his wife definitely that the baby could not be spoiled at this age, pointing out that he could quiet the baby by holding her when neither the mother nor grandmother could. Mr. J. also felt his wife should offer the baby formula more frequently so she could get more rest, should take the child out more frequently, and should not over-dress her. In all, the paediatrician felt his attitude was more 'rational' than was his wife's.

The paediatrician summarized his contact with the statement that although the mother had had a very stormy early period at home, she had made a good adjustment and was doing a much better job than she herself thought. He felt that the chief disturbing factor during the early weeks was the presence of the maternal grandmother. After the grandmother had returned home, Mrs. J. seemed more relaxed and at ease. Also the family had bought a small house in the suburbs, and were looking forward to moving into larger quarters.

DEVELOPMENTAL HISTORY

(a) Introduction

When Sandra was six weeks old, the J.s moved to a small house in a development on the outskirts of the city. The house contained two bedrooms, living-room, dinette, kitchen, and bath. There was a small front yard, and a backyard which the J.s fenced in. Although the street in front carried no 'through' traffic, there were a fair number of delivery trucks and residents' cars passing daily. The 'neighbourhood' consisted of about fifty houses identical in basic structure, which were occupied mainly by 'white collar' workers of middle class socio-economic status. The J.s, by virtue of their education and university connexion, were intellectually though not economically superior to their neighbours, and continued to associate socially with other graduate students and young faculty members. They kept up their social life after Sandra's birth, though arranging for a 'baby sitter' sometimes presented difficulties. They also kept up their interests in the theatre, attending plays and concerts. As Mrs. J. explained later, she felt that the marital relationship came first, and children had to fit into the parents' lives and activities.

Mr. J.'s classes and part-time teaching required him to be at the university from 9 a.m. to 5 p.m. Monday through Friday, and on Saturday mornings. However, he was able to avail himself of the university holidays, and could then devote a larger amount of time to his family. Mr. J. was reported to be fond and proud of Sandra, but did not participate much in her actual care. As he also did not participate in the housework, and as Mrs. J. had no household help, the routines of the home devolved almost entirely on her. Mrs. J. stated frankly that she did not care for housework, and tended to do as little as possible. This was corroborated by a visitor to the home who reported that the house was not attractive, and Mrs. J. apparently was not interested in it.

When Sandra was six months old, Mrs. J. suffered a severe 'nervous breakdown', which necessitated her hospitalization for three months. Her hospitalization followed another visit from her mother, and was precipitated by an intense paranoid delusionary attitude toward her husband, which expressed itself in fears of being poisoned. Treatment revealed that Mrs. J.'s relationship to her mother and poor heterosexual adjustment were basic to her sudden 'break'. During this period, Sandra was sent to stay with her maternal grandmother. Little is known of this household beyond one statement from Mrs. J. to the effect that she thought her mother's general attitudes were similar to her own, because neither believed in strict schedules. With electro-shock treatment and psychotherapy, Mrs. J. experienced a fairly rapid recovery, and was able to resume her normal life. However, as a result of the shock treatment, she forgot most of the details of Sandra's birth and first six months of life. When Sandra returned home at nine months, Mrs. J. hardly remembered her.

Despite Mrs. J.'s post-partal difficulty, the J.s continued with their family planning. When Sandra was two and a half, Mrs. J. became pregnant. She again experienced severe nausea through the first trimester, and was concerned over the possibility of a recurrence of her emotional disturbance. As Mrs. J. felt that fatigue had contributed to her previous post-partal difficulty, and as the extreme nausea was quite debilitating, she spent a large part of each day during the early months of her pregnancy resting in bed.

*　　*　　*　　*　　*

The following described patterns of health, general development, feeding, sleep, elimination, response to guidance and discipline, and social development, are based on information obtained from the paediatrician's, psychologist's and social worker's contacts, and the mother's report by questionnaire. The various records showed good agreement, and are therefore presented as a composite picture of Sandra during her first three years.

(b)　Health

Sandra's health during this period was quite good. Her medical history for the three years is notable for the absence of any severe illness, or recurrent minor ones, such as colds, stomach upsets, or trouble with teething.

Weight and Height by Age

Age	Weight	Height
Birth	7 lb. 7 oz.	20 in.
$5\frac{1}{2}$ weeks	9 lb. 6 oz.	$21\frac{1}{2}$ in.
9 weeks	11 lb. 12 oz.	$22\frac{1}{4}$ in.
$15\frac{1}{2}$ weeks	15 lb. 5 oz.	$24\frac{1}{4}$ in.

5 months	18 lb. 7 oz.	$25\frac{3}{4}$ in.
6 months	19 lb. 8 oz.	$26\frac{1}{2}$ in.
9 months	22 lb. 8 oz.	$28\frac{1}{2}$ in.
$10\frac{1}{2}$ months	24 lb. 3 oz.	$29\frac{1}{4}$ in.
13 months	25 lb. 11 oz.	$30\frac{3}{4}$ in.
16 months	28 lb.	$31\frac{3}{4}$ in.
24 months	33 lb.	$34\frac{3}{4}$ in.
27 months	35 lb.	$35\frac{1}{2}$ in.

Medical History:

5 months: Dry, cracking eczema on lower extremities with small patch on forehead—? wool dermatitis. Rx: lanolin ointment.

9 months: First inoculation of triple toxoid (diphtheria toxoid plus tetanus toxoid plus pertussis vaccine) 0·5 cc.

10·5 months: Second inoculation of triple toxoid 0·5 cc.

13 months: Third inoculation of triple toxoid 0·5 cc.

16 months: Scattered seborrhoeic dermatitis on back of neck—? egg allergy. Rx: treat with ointment.

28 months: Cold, followed by fever of 103·6°. Diagnosis: ? upper respiratory infection or roseola.

38 months: Smallpox vaccination

(c) General Development

Specific data about Sandra's general development are somewhat sketchy. The mother's amnesia following her shock treatment prevented her recall of events during Sandra's first nine months, and in her subsequent reports by questionnaire, Mrs. J. tended to answer questions regarding development from the point of view of her philosophy of child-rearing, rather than in terms of the child's actual behaviour. The major events in her gross motor and verbal development were:

3 weeks	Follows moving objects with eyes
4 weeks	Lifts head
6 weeks	Smiles, holds head well
7 months	First tooth
9 months	Begins to creep
11 months	Pulls to stand
13 months	Walks alone. Begins to feed self
14 months	First word
24 months	Single words, jargon

30 months	Combines words
36 months	Sentences. Undresses self, some dressing
38 months	Feeds self well

Sandra was next seen by the rooming-in staff at fourteen months. She bore a distinct physical resemblance to her mother, both in features and colouring. She appeared as a large, husky, blonde baby, attractive in a sturdy way. The impression of 'huskiness' was increased by the way she was dressed, in a red cotton dress which was quite long, and heavy brown shoes which did not harmonize. She was walking freely, but not talking, though she vocalized frequently with a grunting sound which did not seem particularly gay or happy in tone. She was examined on the Cattell Infant Intelligence Scale, obtaining a mental age of 13·4 months. There was nothing in her general behaviour toward the testing to indicate that her capacity was above the obtained low average rating. It required much encouragement and coaxing to get her to carry out the various tasks, she showed little curiosity or alertness, and at no point did she enter actively into the situation. She had only one word, 'bye-bye', so that her verbal development scored at eleven months, slightly below other abilities. Mrs. J. recognized this with the comment 'We don't think she's very advanced'. She went on to add 'She tries to repeat words after me, but is so embarrassed when she can't. Also, it doesn't seem to me that she's as eager to do things for herself as most babies I know. However, we haven't tried to teach her anything'.

Sandra's development continued at this low average rate. During the second year, Mrs. J. tried to teach her a few words so that she could 'show off', but Sandra could not repeat them accurately, and Mrs. J. abandoned the attempt. At twenty-six months, she had only a few single words, but had developed a flow of jargon. Psychological testing was not successful, as Sandra was somewhat negativistic and almost completely disinterested in the Merrill-Palmer materials. The impression obtained on the basis of the few items she did carry out was that her general development was at about twenty-four months, again a rating of low average. Her motor co-ordination was precise, but methodical and slow. Sandra still appeared large for her age, and quite sturdy. However, her fair, curly hair and large blue eyes gave her an appealing and attractive appearance. Again the mother expressed herself as recognizing the fact that Sandra was not talking as much as other children of her age, adding that she and her husband regarded her as an average child. Mrs. J. said she did not believe in trying to 'push' her or teach her, but that she read to her, and tried to get her into contact with children her own age in the hope that her speech would improve. With this latter point in view, Sandra now entered nursery school. Mrs. J.'s relaxed approach to Sandra's development was evident in her attitude toward the child's test performance. The mother did not try to encourage her beyond the point where it was apparent that the upper limit of the child's capacity had been reached; neither did she apologize for her, or excuse her failures on the grounds that she could do similar tasks in other situations.

Sandra's speech improved considerably during her third year, though she was still quite non-verbal when seen at thirty-eight months for psychological examination. According to the mother, she had begun to talk with her contemporaries around thirty months of age, but had only recently begun to use sentences and would not repeat anything by rote. Sandra's sturdy appearance persisted. She had long braided blonde hair; this was something of a nuisance to both Sandra and her mother, but was not cut because Mr. J. liked it and insisted that it be kept long. Although no particular item of her dress was unusual, she managed to appear somewhat dowdy. She was dressed in dark brown, with heavy, scuffed brown shoes, a brown plaid skirt which was too long for her, and a clumsy brown sweater. Her general approach to the testing situation was slow and methodical; she was rather unspontaneous, and talked little. She was given the Merrill-Palmer Scale, obtaining a mental age of thirty-five months, and rating as low average. All verbal items were refused, but judging from Sandra's spontaneous speech, there was no marked discrepancy between verbal and other abilities; rather, her general rate of development was somewhat slow. By three, Sandra was able to undress herself if her clothing was not too complicated and could put on her pyjamas, overalls, jacket, shoes and socks, with some errors (e.g. both legs in one pyjama leg, shoes on wrong foot). She would work a zipper, but was just beginning to use buttons.

The mother expressed herself again as recognizing that Sandra was no more than average and possibly slightly below. She commented that Sandra resembled certain members of her husband's family, particularly his sisters, who were 'charming and lovely people, but not very bright'. She said that recognition of Sandra's slowness had been difficult for her, as Sandra played frequently with children of other university friends who were bright, and it was important to her that Sandra do well. However, she and her husband found consolation in the fact that she was pretty and happy. As Mr. J. expressed it, 'She has blonde hair and blue eyes and doesn't need to worry'. Looking back over the three years, Mrs. J. felt Sandra might have shown more accomplishment if she had tried to teach her words, nursery rhymes, or 'tricks', but 'It wouldn't have been her rate'. She did plan to teach her to read and write and to ground her in grammar, but not until such time as she felt it was appropriate.

(d) Feeding and Diet

0–3 weeks:	Completely breast-fed.
3–9 weeks:	Breast-fed with complementary formula:

               whole milk   4 oz.
               water   1 oz.
               cane sugar   2 teaspoons
               Cough medicine 6 drops and orange juice, 2 teaspoons, added daily.

9 weeks:	Weaned. Formula 6 oz. 5 times a day:

               whole milk   25 oz.
               water   5 oz.
               cane sugar   4 teaspoons
               Baby foods (cereal and fruit) added.

15½ weeks:	Formula changed to:

               whole milk   28 oz.
               cane sugar   3 tablespoons
               Baby foods (vegetables and soup) added.

5 months:	Changed to whole milk. Egg and potato added.
8 months:	Chopped foods begun.
12 months:	Baby foods discontinued.
13 months:	Suitable family foods begun (not specified).
2 years:	Chopped foods discontinued, on same diet as rest of family (not specified).

Sandra was weaned at approximately two months, when the mother's milk became scanty, and the child's tremendous appetite necessitated a change to bottle-feeding. She was held for her feedings until she began a three-meal-a-day schedule at around seven months. Her appetite throughout the first year was excellent; Mrs. J. characterized her as 'thoroughly dependable as an eater, nearly always cleaning her plate'. She seldom refused a food unless it was new to her, and could be brought to eat it with liking if small amounts were offered at recurrent intervals. Her particular likes at this time were fruits, egg, milk, cereal, and orange juice. She had less preference for items such as meats and chopped vegetables, which required more chewing, but refused only chicken and beef heart. At one year, the mother was still following a flexible feeding plan; Mrs. J. fed her at the hours she had most demanded her food in the past, which evolved into the following pattern: breakfast was at 7.30 to 8 a.m., the noon meal at 11.30 a.m. to 2 p.m., depending on the length of her nap, and the evening meal by 5 p.m. or 5.30 p.m. She did not eat between meals.

When Sandra began eating three meals a day, she was fed in a combination chair and table. All of her meals were eaten alone, as the child preferred this arrangement. At one year, she had not begun to use a cup. She first made attempts to feed herself around a year, by trying to grab the spoon. She fed herself 'finger' foods such as crackers and fruit, and began holding her own bottle around thirteen months. For the most part, however, she still preferred to be fed by her mother, who characterized her as 'lazy, easy-going by nature'.

Sandra's good appetite continued throughout her second year, but during the middle of her third year, around thirty months, she became much more variable in her likes and dislikes and food intake, did not seem to enjoy eating as much as she had, and her milk consumption decreased markedly when she went off the bottle. During this period, Mrs. J. at first pressed her to eat when she felt the refused food was good for the child, but during the latter months Sandra became so irritable that she was permitted to leave the table and go and play. By the age of three, this phase was passing, and Sandra was beginning to eat better. According to the mother, she ate what she should, but 'not avidly'. She preferred fruits, sweets, cheese, tuna, salmon, white fish, and vegetables. She was again drinking milk fairly readily. Mrs. J. felt that many of Sandra's preferences were due to her influence, as she herself enjoyed fruit and cheese, and drank 'lots of milk'. Sandra did not care much for meat, Mrs. J. explaining this on the grounds that she was too lazy to chew it. She refused onions, spaghetti, greasy foods, and chilli. A typical day's meals were:

Breakfast:	Milk, orange juice, soft-boiled egg, toast.
Lunch:	Vegetable soup, cheese, apple, raisins, milk.
Supper:	Sliced beef, carrots, cottage cheese, milk.
Between meals:	Ice-cream cone.

She ate more frequently between meals. For instance, she might have her orange juice and milk later in the morning, after the rest of her breakfast, and have fruit or ice-cream in the middle of the afternoon. She was eating all her meals with the parents, and after a brief period around thirty-two months, when she reverted to wanting to be fed, was again feeding herself. For the most part, she fed herself well, occasionally spilling such things as the filling from sandwiches, soup, or crumbly foods such as cake.

(e) Sleep

When the J.s moved into their new house, Sandra was put into a large crib, in a room by herself. She started to sleep through the night around three months, and by one year was going to bed around 7.30 p.m. and sleeping about twelve hours. She was taking a short morning nap of half an hour, and a longer afternoon nap of from one to one and a half hours. Her sleep pattern throughout the next two years was similar. Thus, at three, she was going to bed around 6.30 p.m. to 7. p.m. (an hour later in the summer), and sleeping from twelve to thirteen hours. She took an hour or two-hour nap in the afternoon, depending on how active she had been during the morning.

In general, Sandra's sleep pattern was good. There was seldom any difficulty on going to bed, though infrequently during the first year she would cry briefly and around thirteen months had a period of crying herself to sleep. She was a sound sleeper, varying in sleeping position between side, stomach, and back. She was not disturbed by noises in the household or the presence of company.

During the first two years, she awoke infrequently in the middle of the night. Often, the mother was at a loss to account for this, but at other times, the waking seemed to be associated with being wet, too cold, or too hot. If the child were changed, covered or uncovered, she would go back to sleep immediately. During her second year, she had a brief spell of awakening, apparently afraid. During her third year, at about thirty months, she seemed unusually wakeful to her mother, who thought this was because she was playing more with the neighbourhood children and was more active and fatigued. She infrequently called out or woke from a dream, at which times the mother went in and comforted her. During the third year, when she was about thirty months, she began a period of taking various toys to bed with her, then for a while insisted on having a glass of water on a bedside table. The mother described these habits as 'constantly changing', but 'very definite for a time'. By three years, the following bed-time routine had developed: she was bathed, sat on her father's lap briefly while he talked to her about her day or read to her, then was carried to bed either by her mother or father. She was given raisins or a piece of candy or two, and then both parents said goodnight to her.

During her first two years, Sandra was permitted to stay in her crib in the morning to amuse herself until her parents had had breakfast. Toward three years, when she slept later, Mrs. J. began taking her up immediately when she awoke and called, to prevent her wetting the bed. At three years, if she awoke early, she was returned to her bed or, infrequently, taken into bed with the parents. Her behaviour on awakening was usually cheerful and smiling; she was 'delightful to greet in the morning'. Retrospectively, Mrs. J. summed up her attitudes toward sleeping by saying she had always assumed Sandra would go to sleep when she was put to bed, and had not gone in to her immediately when the child fussed a little.

(f) Elimination and Toilet-Training

Sandra's elimination throughout the three years was normal, with no problems of constipation or diarrhoea. No attempt was made to toilet-train her during the first year. She had, on several occasions, removed her diaper and played with her stool, but this had provoked no reaction in the mother. Around one year, she had begun to show interest in her genitalia, infrequently examining herself while in her bath or when having her diaper changed. Around fourteen months, she was beginning to remain dry for as long a period as an hour. Around eighteen months, Mrs. J. began putting her on a 'tiddy seat' (a small seat fitting over the regular toilet seat), if she had remained dry for a period, but this was somewhat upsetting to Sandra, who did not seem to comprehend the mother's purpose. Also, her bowel movements were so irregular, it was impossible to 'catch' these.

Mrs. J. was advised by her paediatrician to continue with the training, but she felt this would involve forcing Sandra and such emphasis would only be upsetting to both of them, so she abandoned her attempts at toilet-training. From this point on, as Mrs. J. described it, she was 'left completely on her own' and 'trained herself'. By thirty months, Sandra was dry through every third or fourth night, on the others crying in the middle of the night to be taken up or because she had wet. When playing outside, she would urinate or have a bowel movement in her clothing, but if in the house, would go to the bathroom. She indicated her toilet needs with the phrases, 'I have to wet-wet', or 'I have to doo-doo'. By three years, she was almost completely trained, indicating, 'I have to go to bafroom'. She still wet the bed once or twice a week, but as she now did not like to be taken up to urinate, Mrs. J. ignored it, believing 'time will settle this, for she seems to be improving all the time'. Mrs. J. said her neighbours felt it was a 'disgrace' not to have trained her, and her mother thought she had been very dilatory, but she was convinced that early attempts at training would have resulted in 'a battle'.

INTERPERSONAL RELATIONSHIPS

(a) Guidance and Discipline

Mrs. J. expressed herself as feeling that discipline during the first two years of a child's life centred largely around questions of health and safety. With this in mind, she had tried to follow 'the method of letting them tell you when they want to do things'. Her general approach to matters of discipline was expressed in her statement that she 'could be flexible on any given day, but felt that planning for certain goals in socialization was essential'. She felt she was helped in this by her reading (particularly Spock), and by her instruction while rooming-in.

Mrs. J. found Sandra during her first year very easy to handle: 'a pleasure and not a problem'. She felt Sandra was happy and usually reasonable, sensitive to the emotions of others but not nervous or highly strung. The mother characterized her as having the temperament of Mr. J. and his family, 'very easy-going'. Sandra cried only in relation to some definite frustration, such as hunger, when hurt or frightened, or when tired. Mrs. J. tried to handle each situation in terms of the child's need, i.e., feeding her, consoling her, or putting her to bed. Mrs. J. found her affectionate, but independent and self-reliant.

Questions of discipline presented no problem. Mrs. J. considered Sandra too young to have any definite areas of behaviour of which she disapproved, saying, 'She doesn't want or intend to be troublesome, she just doesn't know better'. On the occasions when Mrs. J. had to interfere in her activities, i.e., when Sandra wished to play with some dangerous or breakable object, she tried to distract the child by giving her a toy or talking to her. The following items were forbidden her: glass ash trays, cigarette butts, matches, safety pins, bobby pins (a kind of hairpin), lamps, books, pencils, and telephone. No physical punishment was used during the first year, though on a few occasions Mrs. J. had spoken to her harshly. This usually caused Sandra to cry, which made Mrs. J. feel 'ashamed of herself', because 'her feelings are hurt and she doesn't understand'. Mrs. J. found Sandra quite responsive to this type of handling—'a nice, cheerful little thing who isn't at all stubborn'.

During Sandra's second year, Mrs. J. tried to continue her policy of permitting the child as much freedom and independence as possible. As many dangerous objects as possible were removed from her reach, so that very few restrictions and little supervision were needed. Mrs. J. continued minimizing physical punishment, and had spanked Sandra only for what she regarded as two major dangers—playing with the stove and running into the street.

Although Mrs. J. felt no problem of discipline existed during Sandra's first two years, she found the third year 'terrible'. She described Sandra as struggling for independence, yet inconsistent in her demands for freedom. Mrs. J. described Sandra's behaviour as 'like adolescence', because she remembered her own adolescence as a similar period of conflict. She felt that during the first two years, Sandra had been permitted to do fairly much as she liked, with the two exceptions noted above. In the third year, however, what Mrs. J. termed Sandra's 'desires of ego self-assertion' multiplied, and consequently there were an increasing number of things which Sandra had to realize she could not do. Mrs. J. felt that the year had been a constant process of trying to decide where to set limits, how much influence to exert, and how to handle Sandra's emotional outbursts. She tried to determine what were the long-term goals she had in mind for Sandra, and to deal with situations requiring discipline in terms of these.

Around two and a half, Sandra had begun having tantrums or crying excessively when she could not get her own way. When frustrated, she would burst into tears, stamp her foot, kick the door, or hit at her mother. Mrs. J. tried to handle these situations by talking reasonably to her, but if this was not successful, told her she would be denied something she wanted, or sent her to her room and shut the door. Occasionally, she was spanked. Mrs. J. felt that handling Sandra's tantrums was complicated by the fact that the child was slow in talking and did not understand language, so that it was sometimes difficult to reason with her. On the other hand, she felt that children who talked very early were sometimes at a disadvantage, as they were thought to comprehend more than they did.

The general areas for which Sandra was disciplined were: dangerous situations (crossing street, turning on gas), deliberate destructiveness, excessive whining or tantrums, or deliberate disobedience after being warned. Mrs. J. felt Sandra over-reacted to physical punishment and isolation, so that she did not need to punish her much. Sandra was usually quickly remorseful when scolded, and would bury her head in her mother's lap, saying, 'I love you, Mummy'. Mrs. J. felt that her sensitivity to reproof was not good because she would be more easily hurt, though it did make discipline easier. Because of her resentment of the fears which had been inculcated in her during her own childhood, Mrs. J. was careful never to use threats or arousal of anxiety as a means of punishment. Although at three years Sandra was still in a period of transition from infantile dependence to childhood independence, Mrs. J. found her increasingly reasonable to deal with, and thought that her methods of discipline were effective.

(b) Personal–Social Development

For all practical purposes, Mrs. J.'s actual maternal relationship to Sandra began when the two were reunited following the mother's hospitalization. Mrs. J. could remember so little of the child's early months that she felt as if this marked for both of them 'the beginning

of a new life'. She realized that from now on, her influence on Sandra's social and emotional development was paramount.

It will be remembered from the immediate post-natal data that
Mrs. J. was concerned about the possibility of spoiling Sandra by
giving her too much attention. She stated retrospectively that she had
tried to take a long-range view, and even when the child was small,
had begun to train her to be a happy social adult. Mrs. J. felt that
maternal over-solicitude was bad from two points of view: it gave
the child a feeling of being too much the centre of things, while simultaneously imposing too much adult influence on her.

Because Mrs. J. wished to encourage independence in Sandra,
during the latter part of her first year the child was frequently left to
play by herself, either in her room or outdoors in the backyard. She
sometimes cried sharply when left alone, but would then settle down
to play for as long as two or more hours. She would then fuss, and if
ignored, begin to cry. Her favourite playthings were kitchen utensils,
pans, clothes-pins, cans, bottles, boxes, paper, stuffed dolls and animals, rattles, and balls. The only toys she had which she did not like
were blocks. Mrs. J. felt that Sandra was so happy and self-sufficient
that she did not need to give much time just to amuse her. She tried
to spend most of the late afternoon with her, and when Sandra became old enough to walk well and not fatigue easily, Mrs. J. tended
to make more of a companion of her. By two years, they would go
down town together shopping, or go to the library, etc. Both mother
and child thoroughly enjoyed this somewhat adult relationship. Mrs.
J. explained that she tried to treat her as an adult early by recognizing
her rights and her feelings.

Sandra was extremely sociable from the beginning. Only once
during her first year did she cry at the presence of a stranger; at all
other meetings, she 'looked them over with an unabashed stare', then
went to them readily if they talked to or smiled at her. This continued to be her pattern. By two and a half, she was initially shy on
meeting strangers, but would talk to them after they had been around
about half an hour. She showed no resistance to being left with a
'sitter'—usually a bachelor friend of the parents or a neighbourhood
high school girl—when the parents went out socially, which was
about twice a week.

Sandra's sociability was evident when she was seen at fourteen
months for the psychological evaluation. She ran about the suite of
offices, showing no shyness or insecurity. She approached strangers
in a friendly manner and made an easy social adjustment. On the
whole, she showed much more social than intellectual adaptability.

During her second year, she had more contact with children in the
neighbourhood. However, with one exception, most of these children

G

were older than she. She played quite well with them, up to the point where they would take things from her, and she would respond by pulling their hair.

Her behaviour at the two-year examination was quite similar to that at one year. She came readily into the examiner's office, and later walked up and down the corridor into adjoining offices. This independence of her mother was also evident when she went to nursery school for two mornings a week at the age of twenty-seven months. At her first visit, she entered the room very quietly with her mother, and immediately started pushing a doll carriage around. She became so engrossed in this activity that she did not notice or respond to her mother's good-bye. This became a pattern, so that every morning she went directly to the carriage, allowing her mother to leave immediately.

She tended to play quietly by herself with almost no variation in mood. She appeared very independent of all, approaching no one except the teacher to get help in dressing or toileting, or retrieving something that had been taken from her. She joined the other children for milk and crackers, and for short periods of music or stories, but other than this, she had little contact with them. During her first few days, she would go after toys which she had finished playing with if some other child took them. When told that someone else could play with them, she lost some of her aggression and began looking at the teacher to get permission to retrieve anything which had been taken from her. If told 'yes', she would try to pull it away from the other child. She did not hit other children, and if hit, would look hurt and give up the effort to get her possession.

Her play in general was self-initiated and perseverative in nature. She enjoyed push toys, such as the carriage, or a wagon. She played with a doll, being quite 'motherly' about it. One of her particular interests was in painting. She would sit in front of an easel for hours, covering the paper with long strokes of water-colour. There seemed to be little imagination in her painting, and she was the only child in the group who refused to finger paint, but insisted on the use of a brush.

Sandra was withdrawn from nursery school shortly before her third birthday, because of difficulties in transportation and the mother's pregnancy. In some respects, Mrs. J. felt this was a good thing, as Sandra now was less restricted and supervised in her play than she was at the nursery school, where an adult was always present. Sandra now had to handle by herself situations which arose in her play with other children, and her mother was pleased to note that she was beginning to be more self-assertive in defending her rights.

During Sandra's first two years, Mr. J. took little part in her actual physical care, though he played with her from one to two hours daily. He was described by Mrs. J. as 'a tease and a romper', and from him Sandra learned a 'teasing quality' which Mrs. J. found somewhat upsetting. When Mrs. J. was feeling ill during the first trimester of her second pregnancy, Mr. J. took more physical care of Sandra, and 'got to know her a lot better'. Sandra, who was not used to this much attention from her father, became somewhat obstreperous, but this did not last more than a few weeks. According to the mother, she was very affectionate, and enjoyed the companionship of her parents. She liked to go marketing with her mother, or go visiting. Her play with her father was more active: she liked to romp with him, to be teased, to be bounced on his knee or foot.

By three years, Sandra was quite independent, spending most of her day outdoors playing with other children. She learned to ride a tricycle, liked to swing, to wheel her doll in a carriage, to go for a ride in a bus or car. With the other children, who ranged in age from two to five years, she played simple nursery games, or played with them in her sandpile. Her preferred playthings were her dolls, blocks and tricycle. She had little interest in books. Mrs. J. read to her occasionally, but in general Sandra preferred to look at pictures in magazines. She was fond of animals, particularly dogs, and enjoyed looking at pictures of them.

At the three-year psychological examination, Sandra appeared as a solemn little girl who gave people the impression of 'sizing them up'. Her general tempo of response was quite deliberate and methodical, though she increased in spontaneity as the session progressed. Her free play was constructive: when shown a doll-house with dolls and furniture, she showed interest and understanding of the function of the various articles (e.g., set the table, put the dolls to bed). It was felt that she would probably be more outgoing in a less structured situation, and that in general she was quite socially well-adjusted and self-confident. The mother was aware that she was reacting to the coming baby, about which she had been told, for Sandra would pat Mrs. J.'s stomach and say, 'Nice tum'. Mrs. J. thought that some of the changes in Sandra's behaviour around thirty months were related to her pregnancy. She had observed that Sandra 'hung around her' and seemed more subdued when she rested frequently during the first trimester. However, all the observers who saw Sandra at her third year felt they could concur in her mother's evaluation of her personality:

'If she continues to be the person she is now, she will be very happy. She will enjoy life, she will be herself, she will be free from distrust and selfconsciousness, achieve what she wants, not take herself too seriously. She has a keen sense of humour and the ridiculous. My ambition is to keep her as sure of herself as she is now, keep her as close to us as she is now—then she will never be lonely, misunderstood, insecure. And already she is aware that she must let us have our life and our needs, and that she cannot have everything she wants because others exist besides herself. She is not in conflict with us, and I hope she never will be.'

SUMMARY AND ANALYSIS

Throughout the record, much of the information obtained from Mrs. J. is highly introspective in nature. Her inclusion of data containing criticisms of herself, her husband, and her child, suggests an attempt on her part to evaluate honestly the family picture. Her ability to verbalize her philosophy of child-rearing would certainly seem a reflection of high intelligence, and probably a reflection of her experience in psychotherapy.

In contrasting the ante-natal and post-natal data in this record, one is struck with the inconsistencies in attitude and family relationships reported by Mrs. J. As these contrasts occur before and after her post-partum breakdown, one can only infer that the treatment she received marked a release for her from many of her former patterns of behaviour.

The two dominant themes which emerge in Mrs. J.'s family pattern are those of her relationship to her mother and to her husband. From the evidence available, it would appear that her relationship to her mother was highly competitive and markedly ambivalent. Thus, ante-natally, in verbalizing her philosophy of child care, Mrs. J. stressed the differences in the way she would bring up her children from the way she was brought up, e.g., she would discipline them less harshly; she would supervise them less in their social contacts. However, on the other hand, her unconscious identification with her mother is evident throughout her attitudes toward length of labour, use of anaesthesia for delivery, and reasons for breast-feeding. In the latter instance, her concern as to the quantity of her milk supply suggests that she was quite ambivalent about breast-feeding, but was impelled to do so by her competition with her mother. In view of her over-protectiveness toward Sandra in the neo-natal period (overdressing, keeping indoors), it would appear that she had begun to repeat her mother's patterns in child care also. However, by the time of the child's first birthday, it was apparent that Mrs. J. was carrying through on her own philosophy of child care rather than following her mother's precepts.

There is some indication in the record that Mrs. J. was more masculine than feminine in her interests, and may have felt competitive toward her husband as well as toward her mother. Her lack of femininity is most evident in her disinterest in keeping an attractive home, and in the manner in which she dressed Sandra. In so far as the child's clothing reflected the mother's taste, it was notably plain and unattractive. One can only speculate as to the course which the competitiveness toward her husband evidenced by Mrs. J. in the neonatal period might have taken had it not been interrupted by her breakdown and subsequent therapy.

In the ante-natal data and through the neo-natal period, one received the impression that Mrs. J. focused more on her relationship to the child than on that to her husband. In particular, the content of the paediatric home visits suggests considerable conflict and tension between husband and wife. In contrast, during the contacts with her at one, two, and three years of Sandra's life, one finds little evidence of such conflict. Instead, there is a continuance of their social life and interests together, and a feeling on Mrs. J.'s part that 'the marital relationship comes first'.

The role of Mrs. J.'s post-partum psychosis in this reversal of her attitudes and behaviour is not clear, but from the chronology of events, one can surmise that this crisis and subsequent treatment enabled her to dissociate herself somewhat from her mother, and to change some of the attitudes which had been contributing to her poor relationship to her husband.

Mrs. J.'s ability to carry out her ideas independently of other influences is most apparent when one views her handling of Sandra against the background of cultural expectations in the groups with whom she associated. It will be recalled that the J.s were living in a lower middle class neighbourhood, where Mrs. J. was criticized for her leniency in certain aspects of her rearing of Sandra, particularly in toilet-training. Study of certain child-care practices in the area indicates that Mrs. J. continued to conform, despite criticism, to the more lenient attitudes prevalent in the upper middle class to which she belonged socially, rather than to the more rigid practices current in the lower middle class families among which she lived. Also, from her mother's criticisms of Mrs. J.'s leniency in self-demand feeding and toilet-training, one suspects that Mrs. J.'s practices also represented a break with the more rigid attitudes prevalent in her cultural group when she was an infant.

On the other hand, the cultural expectation for Mrs. J.'s social group, which was composed of graduate students and young faculty members, would be that Sandra should appear alert and advanced. Intellectually, she would be expected to equal the children of her parents' social associates, while exceeding the children in her 'white collar' neighbourhood. Viewed thus, Mrs. J.'s ability to accept the child's low average intelligence without pressuring her or reacting emotionally, is striking.

The position of Mr. J. in this family unit is not clear from the obtained data. In the neo-natal period, he appeared more 'rational' than his wife in handling the baby, and subsequently his reported behaviour toward the child suggested affectionate acceptance. It seems probable that he contributed more actual demonstrative affection in her life, and thus supplemented his wife's more detached attitude.

In retrospect, one sees in this child's life a disrupted neo-natal period, followed by two years of uneventful development. Around thirty months, there then occurred a period of negativism and self-assertion, which occasioned considerable conflict between mother and child. Although one might anticipate some such developmental manifestation around this time, in Sandra's case it was apparently emphasized by her reaction to her mother's illness during the first trimester of the second pregnancy. However, the facts that Sandra's adjustment was improving by three years and that Mrs. J. showed no evidence of recurrence of her former emotional instability, would seem good prognostic signs.

Finally, one sees in this parent-child relationship a situation in which the mother was able to give the child freedom to develop at her own rate in her basic physiological functions, while imposing on her necessary restrictions for her socialization in the society in which she would live. One can speculate that because Sandra was permitted self-demand learning in feeding, toilet-training, sleep, and language acquisition, she was better able to accept discipline for her integration into the family group. Because of her security within her more limited home environment, she was then able to generalize this security to the larger society into which she gradually advanced. The success of Mrs. J.'s balanced views in self-demand rearing is best evidenced by the child's apparent happiness and her acceptance by her acquaintances as a charming and likeable little girl.

5. JOAN

Fourteen months old

INTRODUCTION

The case of Joan R. is taken from a longitudinal, multidiscipline study of excessive infant crying in relation to parent behaviour.

All the infants studied were children of university students living in the Student Housing Project. The study deals primarily with the interaction between the parents and the infant and the assessment of this interaction as an ætiologic factor in crying. Psychodynamic factors influencing the mother's behaviour and the infant's physiologic responses were studied. A description of the mother's handling of the infant was obtained from interviews with her, from observations of her behaviour during her clinic visits, and home visits by a paediatrician and visiting public health nurses.

The form, intensity and duration of the mother's behaviour and responses to the infant and the infant's reaction to human contacts and other environmental factors, both in the home and in the clinic, were investigated.

In the clinic the babies' responses to certain situations were noted and at this time physiologic measurements were made. Psychological evaluation of the parents and of the infant at various intervals contributed to this study. In addition, the mother of Joan kept a daily record, including the times of all feedings, the baby's behaviour and also her own affective feelings in regard to her daily life.

After Joan was weaned, her mother kept up a daily diary, most of which was concerned with her relationship to her husband and her evaluation of the reflection of this on the baby.

CASE SUMMARY

Family History

Joan R.'s case is presented as an example of a baby whose mother has been distressed because of her infant daughter's crying. At the time of Joan's birth, her parents had been married two years, and had been living in this community about one year. Mrs. R.'s background is Italian Catholic while that of her husband is Anglo-Saxon, with fundamentalist religious allegiances.

Joan was three weeks old when we first saw her. At that time her father was a student at the university and the family lived on $120 a month from the G.I. Bill,[1] plus savings of about $2,000.

The R. family lived in a housing development provided by the university for married students, consisting of a closely arranged series of war surplus army barracks converted into student apartments. The R. home was a typical student apartment in which the doorway goes into the kitchen, which is separated from their living-room by a small partition. There was one bedroom and a bath. Mrs. R.'s home was exceedingly attractive and decorated in excellent taste. When visited by the psychiatrist, it was scrubbed clean and was neat as a pin. Not a single piece of furniture was out of place, not a speck of dirt on the floor.

In June, 1951, when Joan was about six months old, the father got a half-time job with a business organization, becoming full-time after graduation in August. He is at present employed there in a supervisory position making $400 a month. In November of 1951 they moved from the student housing development to another low-cost housing project in another part of the town.

Mrs. R. is a short, dark-complexioned brunette who looks her chronological age of twenty-five. Her face is pocked with scars of *acne vulgaris*, giving her skin a reddish, mottled appearance. In the interview situation she was obviously anxious and cried easily and repeatedly. However, she related well to the physician and was likeable and affable. Mrs. R. grew up as the middle child of three siblings. There was a brother five years older and a sister one and a half years younger. The family lived in an Italian community in another part of the country and were surrounded by Italian friends and relatives. Her father died when Mrs. R. was three, her mother when she was twenty-three. Mrs. R.'s earliest memory is of her father's death. He came home with a cold, stood in a draught while looking out of a window and the next day became worse. Mrs. R. was sent downstairs and her next memory is of her mother screaming. After her father died, there was little money and her mother had to work. Mrs. R. was cared for by her grandparents next door. All the money and affection given her came from her grandparents, for the mother was working and had little time or money to give to her children.

Her mother was described as being very efficient and a good housekeeper, though she used to complain of having been very sick and depressed during her pregnancies. She was never affectionate and never cuddled Mrs. R., whose chief playmate was her younger sister. When she and her sister played together, they had 'pretend teas'.

[1]The colloquial term for the government programme which provided various benefits for veterans of World War II. These benefits included financial assistance for further education.

They would often play 'grown-up' and would play 'house'. In doing so, Mrs. R. used to play the mother and the little sister would play the baby. Her older brother teased her frequently in order to make her cry and only then would he stop.

Her memory of her grandmother is of a person who constantly told her what to do. She said that she used to let what grandmother said go in one ear and out the other. However, grandmother became annoying when she constantly harped on things.

Mrs. R.'s education stopped with high school. She made 'A's at first in grade school, but 'C's in high school. She remembers being fond of an eighth grade teacher, but was afraid to admit it then because of her fear of being teased. When she started going with boys at about age sixteen, she was 'fickle'. She did not go to many of the high school parties because they seemed childish to her. She was 'smart alecky' and thought that she knew everything. She liked to dance, but has not danced much since marriage.

Her acne began during adolescence, but subsided completely during pregnancy and returned post-partum. Her physical health is good except for occasional constipation and headaches.

Psychological Report on Mrs. R.

(15th April, 1951). The tests administered were the Rorschach, Thematic Apperception Test, Word Association Test, and the Draw-a-Person test. Mrs. R. made an easy, casual, informal relationship with the examiner and expressed less concern about what was happening to her baby while she was being tested than any of the other mothers seen. Her attitude toward the tests seemed matter-of-fact, but she tended to become somewhat defensive when asked about her associations and could not respond freely in accounting for the possible origin of her associations.

She appeared to be maintaining her equilibrium through fantasy and compulsive defences, but much of her emotional energy was channelled into fantasy and found no outlet in her relationships with people. She tended to become anxious and to retreat from affect-arousing situations. Affect seemed to be frightening to her because of its sexual connotation. She was confused about and reluctant to accept her sexuality. She felt a good deal of hostility toward men and conceived of heterosexual relationships as dangerous and precarious. There was some slight evidence that she felt unacceptable as a wife-person and was preoccupied with the threat of desertion by her husband or with his inability to satisfy her dependent needs. She had not realized any differentiation from her parents and had strong positive feelings toward her father and a mixture of rebellion and passivity in her attitude toward her mother. She seemed to anticipate criticism or punishment from mother-persons, and it was speculated that her own mother was the strong controlling force in her childhood.

There was no significant clue in the psychological material as to her feelings about the baby, but it might be inferred, from the slight evidence of unresolved anal conflicts and some preoccupation with cleanliness along with her concern about parental attitudes, that she might have some difficulties in handling the child.

Clinically one may say that this is the picture of a mild depression and anxiety neurosis in a neurotic character, compulsive type. Compulsiveness and dependency seem to be the chief ego defences.

Dynamically, she was unable to tolerate her hostility toward the child, and responded to the hostility with excessive guilt and depression. Some of her hostility could be explained by the child being unplanned, by the excessive crying, and by the daughter's interfering with the mother's dependent gratification from her husband. It is speculated that she utilized dependency as a defence against anxiety caused by hostility and her feelings of helplessness with regard to her hostility. It seemed rather clear in the interviews that her compulsiveness partially was an identification with her dead mother as a means of gratifying her dependent needs.

Mrs. R.'s mother was apparently a strong, dominating individual who was rather cold but competent. Love and affection seemed to come from the grandparents. The five-year-older brother was a source of pain because of his teasing and the one-and-a-half-year-younger sister reinforced the patient's own oral needs in the form of sibling rivalry. Mrs. R. recalled demanding that she be placed in the same crib with the sister and that both of them be bottle-fed at the same time. With the father's death, she felt deserted and lost. Her hostility toward men and her sexual anxiety perhaps may have its source in this 'desertion' by the father, and the fact that it probably came at a critical time in the development of her emotional relations to him.

During treatment she saw her psychiatrist in the role of the big brother who teased and of the bad mother who was stern, prohibitive and ungiving. The sexual portion of the transference was apparent but never interpreted to the patient. She presented it chiefly in the form of quarrels and arguments with a man, about which she felt very uncomfortable and anxious.

Psychiatric Evaluation of Mr. R.

Mr. R. was a blond young man, appearing a little younger than his chronological age of twenty-eight. He was of average height and weight, neatly dressed in business suit, shirt and tie, and was superficially friendly and affable. At times he was quite serious, but frequently was jocular and occasionally rather sarcastic in his humour.

He related well, but initially, in great anxiety, he spoke toward the side of the room and in a whisper. He obviously over-intellectualized and presented unconscious material of a sort which one might expect from a schizophrenic patient. However, in his period of therapy, beginning in June, 1951, his anxiety decreased and the unusual fantasy material was discarded for discussion of the more realistic factors in his daily life.

Mr. R. was the middle of three siblings. There is a three-year-older brother and a two-and-a-half-year-younger sister. His mother was a very neurotic, exceedingly religious person, who had stomach ulcers and other stomach trouble and, according to Mr. R., vomited every night. He was steeped by his mother in a fundamentalist religious atmosphere. She was over-protective, apparently seductive, and controlled him through her illnesses. His father was an extremely passive man who, apparently, was completely dominated by the mother; according to Mr. R., father 'just wasn't there'.

His earliest memory was a mental picture of long flowing hair. His mother wanted him to be a girl and dressed him as one. He remembered falling off a tricycle and hitting his head. He and the boy next door used to fight and make up. He never had love for this fellow but they were chums. There were a lot of toys and a lot of soldiers. At age six or seven, he remembers some boys in the back yard, one of whom told a dirty story. The patient's mother called him upstairs and he lied when she asked him about the story. He felt guilty for six months afterwards. At age four or five he urinated behind the fence and his mother saw him and scolded him. At age six he brought a girl home and slid down the pond with her. He recalled that as an adolescent he lay on top of his three-year-younger sister and masturbated.

He joined the Army during World War II, and after discharge had a 'nervous breakdown' manifested by nausea, vomiting, great anxiety, and a need to stay in bed all the time. He had to have his mother lie in bed with him in order to comfort him. The 'nervous breakdown' preceded his present marriage. This illness lasted for less than a year and when he was well he married, in November, 1948. The marriage for both Mr. and Mrs. R. had been quite happy until the baby was born. The only difficulty Mr. R. had had was severe anxiety, nausea and vomiting on leaving his family home one year before the birth of the baby. He was seen for the first time in a routine interview, 23rd March, 1951, when Joan was three months old. In June of 1951, Mrs. R. requested psychotherapy for her husband, which was begun at that time. His chief complaint was a band-like pulling sensation at the back of his neck whenever the baby cried. The father has been seen at once-weekly interviews since beginning therapy, and the dynamic formulations were made from the material of these interviews.

Psychological Tests were made on 1st April, 1951. The tests used were the Rorschach and the Rappaport-Menninger Word Association Test. Following is the Rorschach Summary and clinical evaluation:

Subject's behaviour was characterized by extreme tension and overt signs of anxiety. During Rorschach administration there was progressive deterioration of test responses which was paralleled by overt signs of mounting tension and discomfort. There was a progressive increase in Subject's involvement with the test blots and the loss of distance (responding to the blots as real) was pronounced. During testing he developed a severe headache, perspired freely, and on Card VIII, following his response 'after-birth . . . sure looks messy', Subject became quite ill. Testing was discontinued until Subject regained his composure. His recovery was not complete and he complained of feeling ill at the conclusion of testing. He returned to his home and retired for the remainder of the afternoon.

The mental life of this Subject appears to be dominated by a preoccupation with his sexual conflicts. Sixteen pure sex responses were produced and sexual ideation at the symbolic level was found in numerous other responses. Preoccupation with homosexual impulses accompanied by overt and covert signs of anxiety is characteristic of his Rorschach protocol.

The personality structure follows a schizophrenic pattern. The classic signs of schizophrenia are present in his production and include low $F/\%$, confused sequence, positional determinants, alogical and contaminated responses. There remain, however, personality vectors which continue to support a modicum of reality ties which allow Subject to function marginally in his social, domestic, and economic life. He is able to produce popular responses, can still integrate affective drive with reality (FC) and can show affective responsiveness.

The clinical impression is that of a severe personality disturbance characterized by anxiety and somatization. Schizophrenic processes pervade the personality framework but positive personality vectors yet sustain marginal functioning. Sexual conflict and homosexual impulses appear as strong agents of probable importance in the ætiology of the personality disturbance.

One might diagnose Mr. R.'s illness either as schizophrenia or as decompensating neurotic character, with anxiety of near panic proportions as the chief symptom.

Dynamically, Mr. R. has great dependent needs, both as a fixation and as a defence against great competitive and oral aggressive wishes. He is greatly narcissistic, as manifested by his feelings of masturbation inside his wife rather than real intercourse, also manifested by an extreme sensitivity to any criticism which may imply a recognition of his anal and oral hostility, the expression of which causes him fear of desertion by his mother-surrogates. There is very clear castration anxiety, manifested by dreams and associations to the effect that sexual activity with a woman will result in losing the tip of his penis, also that masturbation will cause an inability to have intercourse. His daughter he thinks of as a living proof to his parents that he has had intercourse; thus his daughter is a great source of terror to him. His dreams reveal his feminine identification and his sexual fantasies about his daughter which are very terrifying and are completely unconscious at this time. He has great fear of looking at the female genitalia and simultaneously a great curiosity about seeing them. He has frequent diarrhoea as a manifestation of his anal hostility and simultaneously a wish to gratify a mother-surrogate. There is sibling rivalry manifested toward his daughter and much anxiety about his death wishes toward her, some of which approach conscious awareness.

Psychogenetically, Mr. R. was reared as a girl. His mother controlled him through vomiting and sickness, making him feel as if he had caused it by his various misbehaviours, such as masturbating and expressions of anger and wilfulness. He also was terrified of her and was unable to find any kind of protection from her through his father. There was hatred of his father because of the father's passivity. Mr. R.'s only defence against the terror of his relationship with his mother was feminine identification, compliance, passivity, and dependence. The older brother seemed to be the favoured son and the younger sister seemed to be the favoured daughter, thus reinforcing the patient's inadequacy as a masculine person.

In the transference, the patient was initially very provocative and hostile, but presented this material like a small child. Initially, he treated the psychiatrist as a mother, later as a father-surrogate, and most recently, after seven months of therapy, has been testing his sexual feelings through the presentation of extramarital fantasies to the therapist. The oral aggressiveness and dependency, the castration anxiety and further dependency, and the hostility as a defence against dependency are all quite evident in the transference.

The therapy has been of a 'relationship' type, interpreting almost exclusively the relationship with the therapist and ignoring a great deal of the childhood and the outside world, including his family and his job. There seems to have been a considerable diminution in anxiety and panic. The patient now talks quite freely with considerably less anxiety and less 'free-floating hostility' and is able to face the therapist and speak quite openly and frankly.

PRE-NATAL, LABOUR, AND NEO-NATAL DATA

The parents were married two years before the birth of Joan. They moved to this city after being married one year, in order that Mr. R. might get away from his mother. The pregnancy was unplanned, and Mrs. R. was 'surprised' when she learned that she was pregnant. The sexual adjustment was not without difficulty in that it took her 'six months to adjust'. She had 'inhibitions'. She said that her husband was kind, patient, and nice. On their honeymoon she was afraid and cried, therefore they had no intercourse. After eight months of marriage intercourse became relatively satisfactory in that Mrs. R. had an orgasm 50 per cent of the time. After she became pregnant, she feared that intercourse would harm the baby and in some way would cause a miscarriage.

Mrs. R. started medical supervision of her pregnancy two and a half months after conception. She felt very well during the entire nine months. Her acne was less than ever before. She had little or no nausea. For the first five months she was seen by her obstetrician every month, then every three weeks until seven months, every two weeks until eight and a half months, and then every week. At each visit, weight, blood pressure, and urine-analysis was done. Mrs. R. took advantage of opportunities to learn about baby care. She attended pre-natal classes at the university and at the Red Cross. She welcomed the Visiting Nurse who visited her ante-partum at seven and a half months and eight and a half months. Neither the Visiting Nurse nor the paediatrician ever saw any results from this attendance of classes or gaining of information by reading. Mrs. R. planned to breast-feed her infant. She said she was influenced by 'reading so many articles about the advantages of breast-feeding babies'. There was no particular care given to the nipples pre-natally.

Mrs. R., by seven and a half months, had gained 18 lb., which her doctor said was the limit she was to gain. By eight and a half months, when the Visiting Nurse called, everything was in readiness for the baby's coming. Mrs. R. had gained 20 lb. and was using skim milk in an effort to maintain a low calorie diet. Although she and Mr. R. had previously planned to have his relatives help her on return from the hospital, they had now decided not to have anyone. On both visits the nurse was impressed with Mrs. R's need to be a perfect housekeeper and to have a 'perfect baby'.

Labour was spontaneous and lasted twenty hours. The mother has no memory of most of it because of sedation. Labour started at 4 a.m. on 24th December, 1950. Mrs. R. was at term and the baby in a vertex presentation, right occiput posterior position. Her obstetrician was out of town and had left his patients to the care of another physician. Although he had seen Mrs. R. several days earlier, the obstetrician had not mentioned his leaving to her. Mrs. R. was very upset at first when she called and found her obstetrician was not available. Two days post-partum she said that she had learned to like the substitute physician. Pains were mild at first. The membrane ruptured at 9 a.m. and at 8.45 a.m. Seconal, grains 3, was given rectally. The records show that pains became stronger during the day and at 7.15 p.m. Scopolamine, grains $\frac{1}{150}$, and Morphine, grains 1·6 were given subcutaneously. The baby, a normal female infant, was delivered at 11.59 p.m. The head had presented in a right occiput posterior position, and although an attempt was made to rotate the head with low forceps the rotation did not hold until the forceps could be re-applied. The infant was delivered in the posterior position with a resultant second degree laceration of the perineum. The placenta and membranes were delivered intact. At this time there was a moderately severe haemorrhage with an approximate blood loss of 300 cc. The patient's pulse rose from 80 beats per minute to 110 beats per minute in the hour following delivery. Blood pressure dropped to 76/40. While the haemorrhage was controlled by suturing the cervix and by effecting haemostasis, in the perineal laceration, 1,000 cc. of 5 per cent glucose was started intravenously, this at 12.15 a.m. Five hundred cc. of whole blood was given intravenously at 1.35 a.m. The condition of the patient was satisfactory all the time, although there was a drop in blood pressure.

In eight hours the temperature rose to 99·4 and the pulse to 108 per minute; however, Mrs. R. ate breakfast well and was able to void. She felt fine except for the tenderness of the perineum. Two days later she was allowed to get up for ten minutes and the following day was given bathroom privileges. Mrs. R. stayed in the hospital eight days with her baby.

The baby's condition at birth was excellent and the cry and respiration were spontaneous. Birth weight was 7 lb. 11 oz., and length was 19 in. The first day post-partum, glucose water was given at 2 and 6 p.m. and taken fairly well. The amount was not known. The baby had quite a lot of tracheal mucous. Meconium was passed per rectum. Twenty-four hours after birth the baby was put to breast and nursed fairly well. After that it was every four hours. On the fifth day post-partum the baby was noted to have a hoarse cry. Her chin was red at this time and boric ointment was applied. The baby's birth weight in the hospital was 7 lb. 11 oz., dropped to 6 lb. 15 oz. three days post-partum, and was 7 lb. 5 oz. seven days post-partum.

In the hospital the baby was offered one breast at each feeding and allowed to stay with the mother to nurse, if she wanted, for twenty minutes. Thrush started three days post-partum and lasted fifteen days. It was never severe and was treated by swabbing the mouth with Gentian Violet solution twice a day.

JOAN'S FIRST YEAR

Crying started the afternoon the mother and baby came home from the hospital and for the first week appeared at all times of the day. During this time the baby got from 19 to $21\frac{1}{2}$ oz. of breast-milk in twenty-four hours. The mother seldom responded to the crying of the baby by feeding her immediately, although she frequently inquired of the Visiting Nurse and the paediatrician whether she should do so and told the paediatrician she was on a 'self-demand' schedule. On coming home, Mrs. R. breast-fed Joan, using both breasts each feeding. She nursed sitting up, and after the 2 a.m. feeding the baby stayed awake until 4 a.m. several nights when first home. The Visiting Nurse visited the family the second day they were home and demonstrated a sponge bath and the method of swabbing out the baby's mouth with Gentian Violet. At this time the father was helping in the house. During the first few weeks he cooked, he bathed the baby, he washed the dishes, and he did the shopping errands.

By fifteen days post-partum, the crying had developed into a pattern of from one and a half to four hours each evening when the mother was tired. At times she cried with the baby. Mrs. R. said that the baby cried as if her heart would break. She said that it 'kills us to let her cry'. At night when the baby woke Mr. R. got up with his wife because it made him too anxious to lie awake in bed.

Holding at times comforted the baby. This holding had to be a fairly active process because unless the baby was jiggled or rocked or walked with she continued to cry. This was also true of taking her in the baby carriage. She was quiet when it bounced, but cried when the motion stopped. The mother always held her securely, but not always close to her body. She said that she was afraid to touch or hold her for fear she might cry. To our knowledge she seldom caressed her. At three weeks she told us that she varied the baby's position of sleeping but hadn't thought of the baby's preferences. The father was unable to study at home because of the crying and left each evening for the library, staying there from 7 until 10.30 on most nights. By eighteen days the mother expressed much anxiety to the Visiting Nurse as to whether she was adequately caring for the child, and on the afternoon of the nineteenth day, her paediatrician prescribed phenobarbital, grain 1, to be given the baby each night at five o'clock.

For a week the baby was described as placid and happy daily. The mother described herself as energetic and happy. The baby took a greater quantity of milk, 23 to 31 oz. daily. At this time she nursed as long as one and a half hours, including burping at times. Feeding was given quite regularly every four hours. Ten drops of a multi-purpose vitamin were given daily. The baby at this time turned to follow the parents' voices. She woke between feedings, whimpered, and dropped back to sleep. On the twenty-seventh day, following this week of quiet, the single dose of phenobarbital given each afternoon was discontinued. The baby was fussy all day. She 'balked a bit at nursing' and Mrs. R. complained of being tired. The baby only took 20 oz. of milk that day.

At four weeks, Mrs. R. and Joan came to the clinic. Mrs. R. said she had noticed the baby sucking her thumb. She told the psychiatrist that Joan was not eating as much or crying as much. After the last evening feeding it took Mrs. R. about two hours to quiet the baby. After Joan had slept one or more hours, at this time, she woke and the mother nursed her again for two or three minutes. The baby then slept the rest of the night. Joan was awake and quiet during the day, but Mrs. R. was afraid to pick her up or play with her for fear she might cry. Mrs. R. had clear-cut physiological symptoms of anxiety when the baby cried at this time. The mother was observed nursing the baby. She held her firmly, but not too warmly, not holding the baby close to her body. The baby nursed vigorously nine minutes on one side and seven on the other without any stimulation by the mother. During this visit, Mrs. R. felt that she had been criticized by the medical personnel because she didn't 'cuddle Joan' enough. The next day was one of mild chaos. Joan cried all day long. Mrs. R. felt tense and upset, overworked and 'very unhappy'. In the afternoon the Visiting Nurse visited in the home. She found Mrs. R. very 'bothered by the crying'. Mrs. R. also compared Joan unfavourably with the neighbour's child of the same age. The baby was dozing in a car bed in the living-room. The Visiting Nurse demonstrated preparing and feeding cereal. Joan took from three to four teaspoonfuls of dry cereal, which had been moistened with milk, willingly and fairly well for the first time. Mrs. R. watched and then said, 'Tomorrow she won't do this for me'. Two days later the baby ate less and regurgitated most of her 10 p.m. feeding almost as soon as she had taken it. The mother was very tired. On this day the baby refused to take any cereal.

This pattern of fussing, crying, and vomiting continued, more frequently in the evening, although also occasionally in the daytime. The baby sometimes acted as if hungry one and a half hours after feeding. The mother was annoyed with the interruption of her work or relaxation. Mrs. R. said rather defensively that her husband could comfort the baby equally well. The crying went on seven days a week, and Mr. R. helped her during the week-ends. We can detect no change in the crying at week-ends. Mrs. R. commented about how important a regular feeding schedule was to her, because irregularity interfered with her housework. She exhibited considerable anger and guilt by crying when she said this. Although upset by the baby's crying, Mrs. R. avoided nursing the baby at that time—('nursing is a nuisance and tiresome')—especially since she is afraid to lie down for fear of smothering the baby. The stools, which had been originally, on coming home, five to seven times a day were now appearing three or four times a day. Over the next week there was considerable discussion as to whether the baby vomited because of a specific food such as cereal or banana, and different fruits and cereals were tried and discarded. Vomiting occurred at one single time in twenty-four hours or less. It was always immediately after being fed. It was usually after the evening meal. Vomiting on occasion was preceded by several hours of crying and on others was followed by hours of crying also. One example at six weeks and six days is, 'Joan was just fine again during the day, but became quite fussy from 7 until 10 and was unhappy even when we held her. I put her down for the night at 10. She awakened at 10.20 when I burped her, then she threw up while she was sucking for a few minutes'. By the time of Joan's six-weeks' visit to the clinic, the mother was able to express her annoyance with the baby's crying and the fact that she wasn't able to comfort the baby.

We know that the husband studied most of the time, was home from 6 to 7.30 for supper, and went to the library after that until 10.30 or 11. He came home while Mrs. R. was still feeding the baby. This quarter he got very high grades. Occasionally, the R.s took a ride and the baby usually slept in the car. Once in a while on Sunday night they went to a movie but, on one occasion, at five weeks and six days, 'Joan was very sweet all day, but fussed from 7.30 until after 9. We wanted to sneak away to a movie tonight and she must have sensed it, the little dickens'. We can see at this time that the mother's major efforts were directed not too successfully toward caring for her baby who cried, whimpered, woke, regurgitated, and often refused to be comforted. If the baby went to sleep in the evening, their next-door neighbours would care for her while they went out for a short time. If the baby fussed they felt they must not leave her. Mrs. R. was more or less confined to the small house and had few visitors because she was 'always tired and not sociable'. The next-door neighbour had a son three months older than Joan who never cried, and on many occasions we have noted the mothers comparing their children, usually in a very unfavourable way for Joan. This neighbour treated Mrs. R. like a younger sibling and directed her or criticized her in a rather bossy way. We were increasingly aware of the lack of success experienced by these parents in the first six weeks, and of their growing annoyance and discouragement with their child. We are also aware of how little Mrs. R.'s dependent needs were met during this very stressful period and how great was her anxiety. She repeatedly came to the clinic or called on the telephone for reassurance about things which she already knew.

A visit by the psychiatrist at seven weeks was planned a week before. As the time approached, Mrs. R. became more anxious. She slept poorly and on the day previous to the visit became very tired and apprehensive. The baby showed increased crying, 'not sleeping an hour all day and that fitfully', and vomited twice in twenty-four hours. The baby also had four bowel movements, an increase over normal. The baby acted as though she wished to nurse every two and a half hours, and also developed 'a new habit of whining before dropping off to sleep. She whines, naps a few minutes, wakes up, and whines more'. The Visiting Nurse who saw the baby at this time quieted her to the point of sleep and put both the mother and the baby to bed, after taking the baby's temperature, which was normal. This was in the middle of the afternoon. At five o'clock the phenobarbital was given to the baby. The next day, both mother and baby were better and maintained a calm appearance for the psychiatrist, although the baby nursed oftener than usual.

On 16th February, 1951, baby's age seven weeks, the psychiatrist reported:

'I had a ten o'clock appointment with Mrs. R. to visit her in the home. This time was chosen because this was the time that she bathed the baby. As she bathed Joan, I sat a little behind the mother. While she bathed her, she talked repeatedly and continuously in a tender, coaxing, reassuring fashion to the child. She said Joan was upset last night. When she bathed the head Joan began a squealing, piercing cry, with much waving of the arms. This was done before the baby was undressed. As soon as she stopped, the crying stopped. The mother did not talk to me unless I questioned her. She placed Joan in the tub and Joan squealed loudly again with a flushed face. The crying stopped immediately when the mother began rubbing the abdomen and chest with soap and water. She talked continuously to Joan, smiled, and was very pleasant. Joan was quiet, but moved continuously and awkwardly as an infant does in holding its head up for the first time. She dried Joan whose eyes were open, and who was moving about awkwardly, but was quiet. When she put Joan on her back to put on her diapers again, she began the piercing squeal and crying. Mrs. R. dressed Joan rapidly and skilfully without hesitation, without clumsiness, and without apparent anxiety. As soon as she picked Joan up and held her on her shoulder, Joan stopped crying. She cried again when the mother laid her on a blanket. She then laid Joan on the scale and Joan began crying again. Mrs. R. explained to me that Joan cries every time she is put on the scale. She comforted Joan again by holding her on her shoulder and the crying stopped immediately. She put Joan crosswise on her lap and Joan cried again. She gave her some vitamins with a dropper and the crying stopped immediately. As soon as the vitamins were stopped, the crying recurred. She then nursed Joan in front of me, and the mother had no apparent embarrassment about exposing her breast in my presence. The baby nursed rapidly and stopped crying as soon as the nipple was put in its mouth. The baby was not held closely, but in the lap. It gagged and cried. The mother was patient and when Joan choked she sat the baby up and talked to her. Joan then stopped crying, and was returned to the breast.

'Mrs. R. commented that Joan usually does not cry when the diapers are changed but yesterday and today there has been this high-pitched piercing cry. Joan went to sleep while nursing and the mother flicked the cheek rather gently with her finger. I asked her how she felt about my coming today. She said that last night she felt a little anxious but not today. At this point she said she didn't dust because she knew that a man would not notice any dust. She did make a special effort to wash the dishes before I came, however.

'After seven or eight minutes Joan went to sleep again. Mrs. R. thumped her feet with her finger rather sharply. She coaxed her and thumped her face and neck but still she did not wake up. Joan slept most of the second half of the first ten minutes of nursing. She said that if Joan falls completely asleep she wakes up in about half an hour and wants to eat again. After ten minutes of nursing the baby was completely asleep. The mother held her in a sitting position, patted her back, tickled her, moved her chin, and seemed quite persistent in trying to get her to wake up. She spent six minutes trying to waken the baby. She then stopped and let her sleep. She once held the baby's eyes open and accused her of pretending and playing possum'. She then weighed her and she slept on the scale this time: she had taken 4 oz. of milk. On being picked up from the scales Joan was awake but did not fuss. The mother held the baby over her shoulder and patted her on the back. She then put her to bed.

'Back in the living-room Mrs. R. said that she was tired because the baby was up all last night. She feels better today because the baby feels better, but she was worried a lot at the time. She had the Visiting Nurse and also called her paediatrician. This is the first time the baby has ever been sick. She was afraid because she thought the baby was in pain; however, she herself did not feel frightened for she knew that it wasn't serious. I asked her what was different in today's bath and she said there was no difference.

'My conclusion about this home visit was that I obtained little, if any, significant material; that the mother was tense, constrained, and by no means was this a normal and natural day for her. I believe that the more controlled environment, such as the office, is a better gauge of the mother's and infant's behaviour.'

When Joan was nine and a half weeks, Mrs. R. reported that the wakeful period was between 6.30 and bed-time. During this time she has to be held and will scream if set down. The crying occurs at no other time of day. Mrs. R. admitted overt annoyance at Joan's interference with her dinner hour and evening relaxation. She again expressed concern that Joan was not on a schedule.

At ten weeks, four days, early morning waking started (2 to 4 a.m.). The school term was over and the parents had planned to drive to visit the father's uncle in a neighbouring state at the end of this week. When Joan was eleven weeks and two days old, the mother seemed excited, at her visit in the clinic, about the prospects of travel the next day. Mrs. R. also complained about the night waking and the fact that the baby needed to be fed then, although she refused to eat solids in the daytime. Mrs. R. also revealed great loneliness, anxiety, and a wish to be cared for and mothered, when she talked to the psychiatrist. The trip was a success, which surprised the parents. Mrs. R. records real delight at the baby's easiness, although she 'needed extra sucking periods' when away from home. However, the trip back in the car was long and crowded. Mrs. R. was tired and the baby screamed for an hour at the end and was very fussy the day following their return.

Two days later the mother developed a cough and fever for five days. She was given penicillin on two days. The mother cared for the baby most of the time at first, as school had begun again for Mr. R. However, Mr. R. stayed at home in the evenings, during which time 'the baby was extremely fussy and seemed unhappy no matter in what position she was held or laid'. At this time, the mother had her first menstrual period since her pregnancy. Mr. R. told the psychiatrist that 'yesterday Mrs. R. got sick' and he knew he had to care for the baby, and the sensation of skin pulling in the back of his neck, which he has when the baby cries, recurred. It is interesting that on three days the baby slept most of the day when the father was away and confined her crying to the 7 p.m. to the 11 p.m. period. On Saturday, as the mother was recovering, and with the father home, she fussed all the day 'sleeping fitfully, never for more than forty-five minutes'. The baby ate less and took less milk, and in the eleven to thirteen week period, which includes these five days of the mother's illness, growth of height and weight, as measured by the Wetzel Grid, showed a falling off. Following the illness, the Visiting Nurse again demonstrated to the mother the feeding of solids. The mother records a week of happiness, with the baby eating better. The weather was sunny and the mother took the baby out in her stroller 'in the sun to the bakery where Joan looked at the clerk and laughed for several seconds'. The baby had fussy periods, but more in the daytime than in the evening, and of a shorter duration.

At fourteen weeks there was a transformation in the mood, attitude, and behaviour of Mrs. R. She said she is over her period of depression; the baby laughs and is better looking. Mrs. R. told the psychiatrist that 'the baby has become a joy more than a chore. The baby is on a four-hour schedule and doesn't take so long to eat and so nursing is not a chore any more'. The mother felt better physically and had more pep. The baby, however, continued to wake any time from 1 a.m. to 4 a.m. most mornings. She also took solids very grudgingly, refusing the greater portion of them daily. Sometimes she cried when they were given. This was a period when Mr. R. was seen for the first time by the psychiatrist, tested by the psychologist, and referred to Student Guidance, seeing both the social worker and the therapist there. After his Rorschach Test he became very distressed. He felt nauseated and came home and went to sleep for three hours on a Sunday afternoon. This week-end Mrs. R. recorded, 'Joan was a wee bit fussy several times during the day. Week-ends seem to excite her more'.

The father's appointment with the therapist at Student Guidance occurred when the baby was almost sixteen weeks. Two days preceding this appointment, Joan woke at 2 a.m. Mrs. R. phoned, telling of her own fatigue and exasperation at the baby's early waking and also at her whimpering during sleep. Phenobarbital was suggested for two nights and Joan slept well, waking at 6 a.m. each morning. At sixteen weeks, Mrs. R. records, 'She certainly is the best little thing all day. She just wakes at night'. Her visit to the clinic at sixteen weeks occurred on the last day before the paediatrician was to leave for two months. Mrs. R. laid the baby, asleep and rather pale, very gently in the crib, and left. As she went out, the baby woke with a start and cried out in thirty-five seconds. Then she looked around, saw the examiner, and smiled three times, kicking gently. The mother's record shows that after the clinic visit and after saying good-bye to the paediatrician, the baby was extremely fussy that evening, from 7 until 10. By that time Mrs. R. was 'really ready for bed'. 'Today for the first time Joan got stuck with a pin. Have been rather careful about that, but guess my hand slipped today. Joan cried for a couple of seconds but soon stopped. Tried to appear nonchalant about the whole thing. Diverted Joan's attention by giving her a toy, then loved her for a minute. Think she'll forget all about it'. That night Joan woke at midnight, but Mr. R. patted her and she quieted soon.

Joan's next visit, at four months one week, took place the day before Mrs. R. and the baby anticipated leaving on a trip to see Mrs. R.'s grandmother and her family, as well as her in-laws. This was also the time the paediatrician, Mrs. R.'s main source of support, had left for two months. Mrs. R. complained to the psychiatrist of feeling lonesome as she did when her mother died. Also about this time Joan started crying when held by strangers and occasionally by her daddy.

It was on Wednesday, 9th May, after some difficulty with Joan's running nose and after several last-minute cancellations by the airline, that Joan and her mother left on a coach plane for their visit. Joan seemed to weather the long trip perfectly. On arriving at their destination, there was much excitement, and it was a very happy time for Mrs. R. Joan seemed to be over-stimulated by the extra attention, but was happy and content. Mrs. R. commented that Joan was completely off schedule. There were a few times when Joan was a little 'cranky' and perhaps was a little restless at night. Occasionally, during the latter part of the stay, Joan would cry unless picked up, and on one or two occasions she was irritable before having a bowel movement, but immediately returned to an excellent humour. On Monday, 21st May, they left by an over-night railroad coach to visit the paternal grand-parents. On that trip Joan was restless all night, and Mrs. R. arrived dead tired with a 'crabby, dirty baby'. They stayed with Mr. R.'s parents four days, during which time Joan was happy and 'perfect', except for a little 'crabbiness' the day before they left for home.

Joan was five and a half months when Mrs. R. returned for her first interview with the psychiatrist after the trip. She reported that she had begun weaning the baby and that the trip was very happy for both Joan and herself. Her only complaint was that Joan didn't smile as much as she would like, and she laughed only with 'excessive stimulation'. Joan had begun to creep, and her nursing time had decreased to five or six minutes. It was at this time that Mrs. R. wanted to talk about her husband and requested psychotherapy for him with the psychiatrist. (The first psychotherapeutic interview with Mr. R. was held on 19th June. It was essentially of the same nature as the original one reported in psychiatric evaluation.) Mrs. R. reported that since her return her sexual life with her husband had been 'normal', with an orgasm almost every time. She reported using a diaphragm despite being a Catholic, and to justify this she replied 'God won't care for my children'.

About a week later, Mrs. R. returned to the clinic and reported her husband feeling jittery and upset and that her baby was cranky, too. She reported feeling very unhappy about her husband's discomfort. It was recorded at this time that Joan was eating only about 63 per cent of a normal caloric intake. Interviews with Mr. R. about this time revealed that he felt very guilty if he didn't help his wife at home, yet he felt very jealous of Joan's crying taking up so much of his wife's time. He was very anxious about the interviews and seemed noticeably upset the day before and the day after the psychiatric interviews, as reported by his wife.

Early in July, Joan was waking in the night, and her parents would spend sometimes an hour and a half walking and quieting her. The Visiting Nurse paid a visit about this time and advised that Mrs. R. arrange to be away from the baby at least one evening or one day a week, and also that the parents let Joan cry without picking her up right away. This was done, and within four days the night waking subsided.

In the clinic, when Joan was six and three-fourths months, Mrs. R. reported that weaning had been completed, and that the home environment seemed to be more comfortable because her husband was feeling better and not so jittery. Following this visit, both Mrs. R. and Mr. R. reported a bad week.

In an interview on 1st August, Mrs. R. reported that life at home had been very unhappy because of her husband's hostility and lack of sexual interest in her, despite her own sexual interest. However, she felt that Joan had been unaffected by the difficulties, for she still seemed cheerful. It was three days later that the husband, feeling reassured by one of the psychiatric interviews, showed a dramatic change in attitude, and became much more friendly and amicable toward his wife. He was able to have intercourse with ease after this. This was only temporary, however; and a few days later he reported another 'fight' with his wife. However, on the same day, Mrs. R. reported in her diary that her husband was better, but still was not sexually interested.

At Joan's seven and a half months' visit to the clinic, Mrs. R. reported that she felt much happier, and that her husband was treating her better. Also, her daughter had been 'good'. Two days after this report of relative tranquillity, the R.s awoke with the house full of smoke because of a failure to light the heater properly. That evening, when the husband was seen in an interview, he felt very guilty, feeling he had almost asphyxiated his baby.

It was about this time, the middle of August, that school was over for Mr. R. Since June he had been working part-time, and after graduation he began working full-time. The latter part of August Mr. R. went on a business trip for one week, during which time Mrs. R. complained in her diary of being very lonely. She reported this at Joan's eight months' visit to the clinic. Joan had been eating poorly and had been irritable, but Mrs. R. had attributed this to teething.

Because the family no longer were students in the university, they had to move from the student housing project, and contemplating this was rather trying for Mrs. R. This, plus the absence of her husband, made her seem 'very dependent' on the paediatrician, as manifested by Mrs. R.'s asking an unusual and apparently excessive amount of advice from her; such as questions about the baby being fed enough, and what did the paediatrician think about moving house, etc.

On his return, Mr. R. reported that he had had a very poor trip. His head hurt, and he was very lonely. After he had been back three or four days, Mrs. R. in her diary reported that Joan was improving in her irritability and crabbiness. Mr. R. reported in his interviews that he still had no sexual interest in his wife and was angry at her. He showed a great deal of hostility toward both his wife and the psychiatrist. Mrs. R., in her diary, however, reported an improvement in the family situation about the middle of September, describing such things as going house-hunting and having a 'perfect week-end'. However, she did report her husband feeling unusually irritable the night before he had his psychiatric interview.

Joan was now eight and three-fourths months. At the clinic Mrs. R. reported that Joan was doing well, and then described her feeding time with Joan, when she talked to her, sang to her, and tried to keep the meal-time as pleasant as possible. Mrs. R. felt that it was very unpleasant when Joan wouldn't eat. She was rather inconsistent about letting Joan feel the food. Sometimes, if annoyed, she was intolerant of Joan's being messy at meal-time and would scold her. However, on some days, she did not feel annoyed by it, and simply tried to distract Joan by giving her a toy. Joan still drank her milk from a bottle, about nine ounces at each feeding, while her mother held her. Occasional attempts to wean her to a glass were unsuccessful.

Mrs. R. played certain games with Joan, such as peek-a-boo and bye-bye. At times she crawled in a circle with her, laughing and talking while doing so. She played these games almost every day. Sometimes she tickled Joan's toes and made gurgling sounds on her stomach to which Joan responded by laughter. Father was rougher, but Joan seemed to love it.

It was in September too, that Mr. R. reported having a need to play with Joan if she were alone, feeling that she might 'feel bad' if she weren't played with. About this same time the family decided upon another apartment, approximately ten miles from their present home. The latter part of September and the early part of October were reported by the parents as uneventful. Mr. R. reported some anxiety about work, fearing that he might forget a name when he had to introduce various people there. They made a short trip, and Mr. R. went fishing one day.

In her October clinic visit, Joan now nine and a half months, Mrs. R. reported that Joan had walked two steps since the last interview and had been sleeping much better, being able to sleep throughout the night with the light out. Mrs. R. was asked about auto-erotic play, and the only type that Joan engaged in was pulling at her navel and occasionally touching her genitals. In talking to the paediatrician, Mrs. R. again asked a great deal of advice, especially in relation to the prospective move.

In her diary on 14th October, Mrs. R. reported that she might be pregnant. This was a source of some anxiety; however, the menstrual period appeared the next day, and she felt greatly relieved. During October, Mr. R. revealed much anxiety in the psychiatric interviews, alternating with considerable anger towards his therapist. Mrs. R. reported 'a perfect week-end' on a number of occasions during this month.

It was the first of November when they moved to their new apartment. Two days before this Mr. R. hurt his back so that he was unable to participate very actively in the move. After the move they didn't like their home. They didn't feel at home. Shortly after the move, Joan was clinging, more irritable, and needed to be comforted more frequently than usual. It was ten days after the move that she developed a cold with a 'runny nose'.

In the November clinic visit, when Joan was ten and three-fourths months, Mrs. R. reported that Joan had been weaned to a cup 'because it seemed like it was time'. She said that she weaned her because she hated the sight of a baby walking around and holding a bottle. Apparently this was a manifestation of identification with Joan and a defence against her own dependent wishes.

During the latter part of November, there were alternate good periods and bad periods for the family, some times when Joan would have a good appetite and would have a good time with her father. However, Mr. R. reported frequently that he would have a 'bad week', and in his interviews death wishes towards his wife and parents began to come out. These wishes were very frightening to him. It was the day after Thanksgiving that Joan became ill with a high temperature, averaging between 102 and 104. She was sick for about three days. Mr. R. felt irritable and had no sex desire toward his wife at this time. The last week in November, he became sick with 'flu and Mrs. R. reported feeling rebuffed by him, and Mr. R. reported feeling rebuffed by her. It was during these last days in November and the first weeks in December that the irritability of Mr. R. and the friction between him and his wife reached its height. In her diary Mrs. R. would report occasionally that Joan would be better, with an increased appetite; and then a few days later would report that she had awakened screaming in the middle of the night. Despite the parental quarrelling, the baby's appetite seemed to be doing very well.

Around Christmas, Mr. R. reported having the same kind of symptoms he had had every Christmas as long as he could remember—that is, abdominal cramps, nausea and diarrhoea, and the feeling of being gypped.[1] His impotence continued during the latter part of December and in January, but the quarrelling between him and his wife seemed to subside so that there was less overt ill-feeling. The first part of January he was offered a job in another state at a salary of $500 per month. He postponed any decision about it, ostensibly to finish his psychotherapy. It was during December that he had little work to do because materials needed in his job had not arrived, but in January the materials arrived and his really active work began.

The last interview with Mrs. R. on 29th February, 1952, revealed Mrs. R. feeling happy with her child, and able to express annoyance and discomfort with her child and with her husband without too much anxiety. She had not cried for months. She reported her husband feeling better and their sexual relationship better but still not what it was before psychotherapy was begun. She stated there had been no difficulties with the baby in several months.

SUMMARY OF PSYCHOLOGIST'S OBSERVATIONS ON JOAN

Psychologist's observations were made on this child at the ages of 18, 24, 25, and 31 weeks. All observations, with the exception of those tests requiring sitting at a table, were made with the child in the crib.

Developmental: The most complete study of development was made at the age of 24 weeks and included Cattell and Gesell scales. The following is a summary of these test results:

Cattell Infant Intelligence Scale

Chronological Age	5·6 months (24 weeks)
Mental Age	7·2 months
Intelligence Quotient	129

[1] A colloquialism meaning cheated.

Gesell Developmental Schedules

Postural Schedule .	. .	30 weeks
Adaptive Schedule	. .	27 (plus) weeks
Prehensory Schedule	. .	31 weeks
Perceptual Schedule	. .	29 (plus) weeks
Language-Social .	. .	Undetermined, but estimated to be normal for age.

Postural and locomotor behaviour showed a marked acceleration beginning at the twenty-fifth week and continuing through the thirty-first week. The twenty-fifth week showed strong efforts to pull to standing and to support body weight in the upright position. At thirty-one weeks the child was taking steps with support.

Behavioural characteristics: The child seemed to depart from the customary exploitation of developing skills through random utilization. As her developmental capacities unfolded, postural and loco-motor in particular, they were employed in apparent service of the child's needs rather than randomly directed. These needs of the child seemed to be for a greater control over the persons in her environment and a need to be alert to subtle changes in her surroundings. Thus, orienting behaviour that maximized impinging stimuli, was consistently and strongly present. Approach behaviour that facilitated interaction between herself and the male examiner was consistently present, and denial of interaction by the examiner's response to her approach behaviour resulted in avoidant behaviour when her approach repertoire was fully exploited.

The child's activity level was consistently high during all periods of observation. She was consistently alert and sensitive to minor changes in the physical and social surrounds. Sleeping did not occur in any observation period. Child was either in self-initiated activity or respondent activity at all times. Much exploratory behaviour was noted and constitutes a prominent characteristic of the child.

The child showed a low tolerance for any action, real or implied, which was suggestive of examiner's separation or turning from the child. In essence, this child seemed more than usually dependent upon the presence of the examiner for the maintenance of a state of satisfaction. A full view of the examiner's face was sufficient to stop crying. Since turning from the child seems to imply the threat of separation, it is felt that this child manifested a need for the examiner's attention and support.

The child was particularly responsive to social stimulation and from the earliest observations exhibited behaviour which served to bring the examiner into a closer relationship to the child. A denial of the child's attempts to bring about a closer contact with the examiner served to produce crying and frustrated, tantrum-like behaviour. She showed a far greater interest in exploiting social interactions than physical objects.

Joan was consistently responsive to the examiner's comforting ministrations. Crying, no matter what the cause, was consistently terminated, usually promptly, by the examiner's talking to the child. Holding the child for quieting was necessary on only one occasion and followed stabbing for a blood sample.

On all occasions in which interaction with, and response to, the mother was observed, this child consistently oriented positively to mother. At no time did she remonstrate against mother's care and handling, and on each occasion of mother's return to the observation room the child would orient positively to mother by smiling or making attempts to approach her.

Summary: The observations picture a child who is extremely active and alert. She shows pronounced developmental acceleration with postural and locomotor control being particularly advanced. She shows marked sensitivity to the social environment and makes consistent efforts to relate herself to it as well as efforts to control it.

The functional utilization of the postural and locomotor skills was so marked as to cause the examiner to question whether or not acceleration in these areas was a reflection of a simple unfolding maturational process, or whether they might not be accelerated additionally through their intensive employment in serving the child's strong needs for postural and locomotor adaptations which reward her with a greater measure of control over the persons and things which surround her.

SAMPLE CLINIC REPORTS

Explanation of Physiological Methods

(i) Observations on face-reddening, tears, and blepharospasm on a four-point scale.

(ii) X-rays were made at least three hours after the last feeding.

    (*a*) A flat plate was taken on arrival.

    (*b*) Following this, 4 oz. of a 1 : 3 solution of barium and boiled water, slightly sweetened, was offered, the baby taking as much as she would without forcing.

    (*c*) A second film was taken immediately at the end of the feeding.

    (*d*) After 45 minutes, three films were taken 30 seconds apart.

    (*e*) The films were taken with the baby prone.

(iii) Eosinophil Counts were made by Dunger's method, using a hypotonic solution of eosin as the diluting fluid. The pipette is shaken *immediately* about fifty times for not more than 30 seconds, and the changer of the haemacytometer filled *immediately*. This is allowed to stand approximately 3 minutes before counting.

(iv) The nasal smears are not fixed. They are stained with Wright's stain. The smear is examined alternately from horizontal to vertical going over the entire slide. Cells are rated as: Loaded, Many, Quite a few, Few, Very few, Occasional and None. When destroyed cells are present, it is designated as debris.

At seven and a half months

Clinic Visit:

> Mother handled baby easily, fondling her as she stood the baby in the crib and handing her a toy. She waited for several minutes occasionally smoothing her hair or giving her a caressing touch. After four minutes she said, 'There now, Joan, I think you're all right', and turned to go. Joan let out one yell and then played with her toys actively.

9.35 a.m.   Nasal mucosa shows very slight hyperaemia and slight swelling of the turbinates. The nasal smear shows no polymorphs and an occasional epithelial cell. There was no startle or cry when her toe was pricked for a blood count.

Isolated

9.43 a.m.   Whining protesting cry at infrequent intervals. She was extremely active moving around the crib and banging her toy. Considerable sucking of toy.

9.51 a.m.   Sits up handling toys, occasionally sucking one. Lies down for about thirty seconds always on abdomen. Is wet at this time.

9.52 a.m.   She kept getting up and down, combining toys, lifting and passing one from one hand or dropping it or hitting it. She kicked with her right foot several times. She began to protest, saying, 'Ah, Ah, Ah'. She then sat up and sucked the toys very hard.

9.53 a.m.   She lay down and began to pound the bed with her right, closed fist. At this moment the examiner dropped her pencil with a clatter. The baby did not seem to startle. Her feet had been held in eversion most of the time and at this moment she was holding them through the crib side. Her cry has become more of a whine at this moment, sounding like, 'Ah, ah, oh, oh, ah, ah, ah', and also it sounds as though she were calling someone. When she is crying at this moment, she is kicking quite violently, and then will stop both for a few seconds.

9.56 a.m.   She is lying across the bed, sucking one toy, and then she handles the other toy and kicks the wall.

10 a.m.   Nasal mucosa shows less colour and less swelling. Smears show no polymorphs and very few epithelial cells. With blood count she let out a cry but was distracted easily.

10.02–   Baby carried in examiner's arms, or sat in her lap.
10.12 a.m.   Joan occasionally puckered up her face particularly after the door was shut. After a few minutes the examiner sat down and played peek-a-boo with her, using a sweater, and she laughed at this until her mother returned at 10.12.

10.12 a.m.   Mother promptly took Joan in her lap and baby sat happily there, occasionally sucking her toy.

10.15 a.m.   Baby cried more with this blood count. Her mother tried to comfort her and held her for a considerable time afterwards. After ten minutes she replaced the baby in the crib. The baby puckered up her face but did not protest and her mother smiled and waved at her and handed her some toys.

Growth failure as before.
Both central upper incisors have erupted.

Mother reports:

Appetite poor while teeth erupting.

*   *   *   *   *

At eight months

Clinic Visit:

Mother looks very tired. Says she has eaten and slept poorly since father away for ten days. Mother very dependent on paediatrician, and delayed a long time talking to the doctor about herself.

9.35 a.m.   Baby puckered up face with separation—objected to restraint of head.

9.43 a.m.   Nasal smears showed quite a few polymorphs and a few epithelial cells. Cried loudly when foot held before blood count and increasingly so when her toe was pricked.

Isolated

9.44–10 a.m. Crying very angrily. Face very red, marked blepharo-spasm and tears.

9.50 a.m.   She lay on abdomen, then rose on all fours and rocked and repeated this, shrieking most of the time. She sucked her toy a lot.

9.52 a.m.   Her nose became obstructed and she was sobbing. When she lies down she throws herself down.

9.55 a.m.   She is completely in a position of flexion.

10 a.m.   Eyes and eyelids very red. She has drooled over a large area of the sheet. She is panting and very apprehensive and wet. Nasal smears show no polymorphs and very few epithelial cells.

10–10.15 a.m.   The baby was held and carried and patted. She clings with her hands to the examiner's shoulder, coat and necklace. She hits the examiner's back at times with great vigour. At times the baby holds herself tensely against the examiner, but at no time does the baby seem to relax in the examiner's arms. On two occasions the examiner attempted to stand the baby in the crib but she began screaming and crying at the very start of the procedure. The examiner at one time said, 'Look at the dog', when she was near the window, and the baby looked alertly and for several minutes followed with her eyes some dogs who were playing outside. The baby seemed fairly contented with the examiner but not truly happy, and she never relaxed for more than an instant. If her foot, or her feet, touched any surface, as for example the crib side, she immediately tried to stand and push up. When she cries, tears are enormous tears, and she is definitely hyper-active here today.

10.15 a.m.   At this time she was sat in the examiner's lap and her toe was again pricked. The baby was screaming as her foot was held, practically crawling up over the exa-miner's shoulder. The mother returned just as the blood count was done and the baby looked at her and

122

went very quickly to her. During the physical examination, the baby appeared quite content and happy as long as she remained in her mother's lap.

Mother reports:

Baby takes solids only at lunch.

Drinks 27 oz. milk daily in bottles. Is held for some of each feeding.

Baby sleeps well but cries out in sleep.

Growth failure.

Haemoglobin 12·25.

Smallpox vaccination on left arm, given with a typical 'take' reaction appearing five days.

* * * * *

CONCLUSION

Joan was an unplanned baby whose arrival was very stressful to the mother and the father. Mrs. R. was a dependent person needing considerable support in her daily life. She had mixed feelings about her unplanned child. Pre-natally she showed increasing need to deal with these feelings by being a 'perfect' wife and mother and having a 'perfect' baby. She became temporarily more confident through reading books, going to pre-natal classes, and depending on her obstetrician and on the Visiting Nurse. She made very complete preparations for the baby. It was a real shock and very threatening for her to find her obstetrician out of town at a time she needed him. He had not prepared her for a substitute physician. She was able to feel that she 'liked' the substitute physician only when labour was over and she was two days post-partum.

Mr. R. also was an extremely dependent person with a severe personality disturbance accompanied by much free-floating anxiety and undirected hostility. The severity of his symptoms at times incapacitated him. He had a great deal of sexual conflict. His daughter he saw as a rival and as a source of great anxiety because of his feelings about her. He felt ill whenever she cried, so much so that he got up at night with his wife to tend the baby. He also studied in the university library as much as he could rather than at home. He did help in practical ways, but over a limited time. He, too, was uneasy with a strange physician, and when he was told about Mrs. R.'s post-partum haemorrhage he was very frightened.

The baby's behaviour on arrival home, which was similar to the behaviour of most new-born infants, was especially threatening to both these parents. Mrs. R. was repeatedly aware of what she considered her lack of success with her child. By three weeks, five days, as she anticipated discontinuing phenobarbital, she felt the baby nursed 'poorly'. By four weeks and one day, she was preoccupied and distressed, anticipating failure in feeding solids to Joan. The mother-child relationship was productive of little satisfaction for Mrs. R. and Joan during the first three months, except for brief times such as the three-day visit to the father's uncle at eleven weeks. Mrs. R. had conflict about feeding and holding Joan, especially during the evenings when she cried. At times Mrs. R. became exasperated because her efforts to soothe Joan resulted in more crying, and with Mr. R. away she had to cope with the crying baby all alone.

In the first three months the baby was observed to respond to a wide variety of stresses by crying, a pattern of behaviour in which respiratory, skeletal muscular, cardiovascular, gastro-intestinal, skin and endocrine systems all participated. In the early months this pattern of behaviour appeared as a relatively undifferentiated response to such diverse stimuli as touch, restraint, noise, pain, noxious fumes, hunger, and need for holding. This crying reaction was more prolonged as a result of stimuli evolving from interpersonal relations than from other types of stress. By three weeks the alterations in functions of certain physiological systems were productive of symptoms for brief periods. I refer to such things as the extreme face-reddening and rash which appeared from six to eleven weeks, and the occasional vomiting from six to ten and a half weeks. Accompanying this pattern of the total reaction, it became apparent that there were alterations in the baby's response to certain stimuli. Certain previously noxious stimuli became less so and others increased in importance. I refer to the startle-reflex with touch, which was marked at four weeks but not present at eleven weeks.

In the first three months physiological components of behaviour were observed to fluctuate more rapidly and over a somewhat wider range than later. In comparing our series of twenty babies during the first four months, Joan ranks next to highest in amount of crying and gastro-intestinal symptoms. She shows next to the highest total gastro-intestinal motility and rapidity in stomach emptying as seen by X-ray. She is in the top group showing nasal reactivity, face-reddening, and weeping. The latter appeared early and was always extreme except on one occasion at fifteen weeks when she cried tearlessly for a short time. Pulse and respiration were relatively stable as judged by our group.

There seemed to be an intimate relation between the degree of maturity and the type of response provoked by certain stresses. It would seem that newly completed functions were utilized often to the exclusion of earlier patterns of behaviour. For example, auditory awareness was present shortly after birth, at which time many auditory stimuli provoked the startle reaction; but it was not until twenty-four days that Joan was observed to follow the parents' voices. At

124

the clinic at six weeks, Joan was asleep in the crib and woke in a few seconds after hearing her mother's voice, although other sounds had been present while she was asleep without any waking. As relative visual maturity occurred at about three and a half months, isolation at the clinic or at home became particularly stressful to the baby, although she would lie in the crib contentedly as long as she could see somebody.

Stimuli evolving from interpersonal relations include positive pleasant stimuli, positive noxious stimuli, and those arising when certain basic needs and appetites are not satisfied. The earliest neonatal mother-child relationships revolved predominantly around eating and holding. In both relationships Mrs. R. was insecure, anxious, and tense, and was unable to achieve satisfaction from her performance. Indeed, her performance was often productive of hostility, frustration and other strong feelings. It has been shown that alterations in feeling states are associated with many body changes in adults. It is postulated that the stimuli in the mother-child relationship which influence the child's behaviour, arise from these body changes in the mother. Thus, the content of Mrs. R.'s feelings was communicated to the baby by tactile, temperature, orienting or postural, auditory, visual and possibly olfactory stimuli. This was also true of the Visiting Nurse and the paediatrician on occasions. As the baby matured, the stimuli involving other sensory systems than tactile and proprioceptive significantly influenced the child's behaviour reactions. It is evident that the mother's transmissions of her feelings involved the way in which she held the baby when breast-feeding and also when comforting her, in her lack of caressing the baby, in her need to cry when the baby cried during the early months, and in her inability to feel comfortable about picking up and reassuring Joan during periods of crying. When Joan was quiet, Mrs. R. also was unable to pick the baby up for fear she would cry. It is also evident that the mother, because of her need to have a schedule, transmitted her feelings by depriving the baby of breast-feeding at times when the baby was hungry. Again we feel the mother communicated her feelings in the way she fed the solids which the baby refused, although the baby took them readily on two occasions for the Visiting Nurse.

Following the baby's discomfort with holding and feeding during the first three months, at later ages the baby was observed to react to stress by calling into play patterns of behaviour appropriate for an earlier age. These patterns of behaviour appeared in those situations that were earlier stressful to her. In returning to these earlier patterns, the physiological fluctuations which occurred earlier appear also to be more extensive in quantity and duration. For example, see clinic visit, ten and three-quarter months.

Response to stimuli productive of satisfaction provoked patterns of behaviour other than the crying reaction. At eleven weeks there was a cessation of crying with head stroking, in contrast to the response of crying to touch with a stethoscope. At sixteen weeks, the baby woke as the mother left and cried out, but on seeing the examiner became quiet and smiled three times. At seven and a half months, the baby's response to her mother's caressing was appropriate behaviour with less nasal reactivity as judged by colour secretion and cells in the nasal smear, although slight turbinate swelling was present. Also at this time there was no reaction to pain stimuli upon having her toe pricked. At various times the prick of her toe for a blood count resulted in no startle or outcry, and at other times she reacted with violent screaming as her foot was held, even before the toe was pricked.

At birth the baby reacted as a total organism to every stress, if she reacted at all, by crying with all its physiological accompaniments. At a later age the same stimuli did not always cause such a reaction. The startle stimulus is an example. As she became older and more mature, there seemed to be a mechanism of selectively responding to stimuli, so that a reaction occurred with some but not with others. The capacity for selective response to stimuli was not present at birth. Feeding, sedatives, sleep, and satisfactory interpersonal relations were some of the factors which appeared to influence the development of this capacity. These influential factors may be of longer or shorter duration, and as such seemed to cause a greater or lesser influence at some times. With Joan the mechanism of selectively filtering stimuli seemed to depend to a large extent on the satisfactoriness of the mother-child relationship as we saw it develop. As we have shown, in the early months this mutually unsatisfactory relationship was productive of crying in the baby.

As Joan grew older, we see variation in the responses to the same stimuli of pain, restraint, isolation and holding. These variations correspond to the relationship between Joan and Mrs. R. at those times, and more basically to Mrs. R.'s reaction to her own personal problems involving her feelings towards Joan and Mr. R. For example, in comparing seven and a half and eight months, we have differences in family stress and feeling. We also see differences in the mother's handling of the child in the clinic. There are differences in Joan's reaction to pain and isolation, also differences in the nasal reactivity, in the cellular content of the nasal smears, face blotching and sweating. Her reaction to pain and to being comforted after isolation also differed. At the time when the family was relatively tranquil, at seven and a half months, all these parameters show little fluctuation; but at eight months with marked family stress they show marked alterations. Another example is the clinic visit at eleven and three-quarter months. In this setting of relative security, the baby was able to tolerate, without crying, such a potentially threatening situation as isolation. There is less reactivity physiologically, with nasal smears showing few cells and no polymorphs and with the eosinophil count decreasing with holding and sleep. One might compare this visit with the visit at nine and a half months, in terms of behaviour, both mother's and child's, rise and fluctuation of eosinophils with or without holding.

6. JERRY

Seven months old

INTRODUCTION

When we came to know Jerry J. he was thirty-two weeks, or seven and a quarter months, old. In connexion with a research investigation of normal infant behaviour, a team consisting of one psychiatrist and two psychologists tried to learn as much as possible about Jerry as he was at that time, and about his development so far. We came to know him and his mother quite well, saw enough of his older brother and learned enough about his history to form a fairly good picture of him, and briefly became acquainted with his father as well.

While the developmental history which will be given is thought to be rather more reliable than many retrospective histories (because the mother was an unusually good observer and because she had kept a diary record of the baby's development), the main contribution we hope to make is a full description of the behaviour of a healthy boy as he responded to a rather ordinary family environment, bringing to his every response his own individual characteristics. Thus, we do not think of Jerry as a model of normalcy, and would not wish to use his behaviour as a standard with which to compare that of others. We do think of him as a thoroughly healthy, well-endowed child who lived in a supportive environment, and whose behaviour illustrates *one kind* of wholesome adaptation possible to babies, subtly different from any other yet like that of many others in some respects.

The reader will be better able to evaluate the material if he knows the manner in which it was obtained. What follows is by no means a full account of our research study, but may suffice for the present purpose. In the course of clinical work with infants and young children, the investigators became increasingly aware of the fact that there is a lack of accurate information about the behaviour of normal infants. While a good deal is known about the regularity of the growth process, and we know the average ages at which certain developmental skills are attained, very little is known about all those aspects of infant behaviour which do not occur with such regularity that they make their way into normative studies. Thus, we know approximately when to expect a baby to sit alone, to stand, to hold a block in each hand or to speak his first words; we do not know much about normal behaviour in the areas of eating, sleeping, interest ranges, expressive behaviours, social communication and the like. Moreover, both where average standards are available and where they are not, very little is known about individual differences among normal children, i.e., about the range of variability that can be encountered among healthy infants. It appeared to us that both a theory of personality development and practical hygiene measures depend on factual information of *what* babies do, *how* they do it and the circumstances under which they do it. Jerry was one of one hundred and twenty-eight babies studied with the aim of making a small contribution to this vast topic.

Our main method was *direct observation of baby and mother in natural circumstances.* In order to feel that observations were as accurate and complete as we could make them, three trained observers simultaneously recorded what went on during the most important phase of the study; observations in the home, however, were usually made by one person at a time. Always, mother and baby spent a period of about four continuous hours with us, in rooms equipped for the purpose. The mother was told to do with and for the baby as she saw fit, and the great majority of mothers soon relaxed and behaved much as one would during a comfortable social visit. Thus, we observed mothers feeding their babies, putting them to sleep, dressing and undressing them, playing with them or leaving them to their own devices, comforting them or 'letting them cry it out', as the mothers chose. They knew, of course, the purpose of our study and rather expected to tell us 'all about the baby'. A large proportion of the developmental history and information about the baby's daily experience was obtained in the course of a continuous, leisurely and thorough interview during those four hours. A few days afterwards the interview was continued in the mother's home, until we felt that we had learned all that this mother was able and willing to tell us. Several procedures were used to objectify our observations of the baby's behaviour. In this context it is of interest only that we administered development tests to all babies, conducted a paediatric examination and obtained some simple measures of physical growth.

CASE SUMMARY

JERRY'S FAMILY

The chief actors of our drama were Jerry's parents, both twenty-four years old at this time, his brother Freddy, aged two years and seven months, and Jerry himself, aged seven months. About a year before Jerry's birth, the parents bought a little house at the outskirts of the town, using a small inheritance for a down payment.[1] Our records describe the home as follows:

'An attractive bungalow on a newly developed street several miles west of town. The street is an isolated one, actually out in the country. All of the homes on it are rather small and new, and apparently there hadn't been time for any landscaping to be done yet. The house consists of five good-sized rooms: living-room, dining-room, kitchen, two bedrooms, in addition to a modern bathroom and large utility room adjacent to the kitchen. Between the kitchen and the bedroom is a hall-way so large that Jerry's full-size crib can be kept in it. It was several minutes before the mother answered the front door. She said that she had been "away in the back".

'I was considerably surprised when she ushered me into a living-room devoid of all furniture except one cabinet, on top of which was a handsome picture of Freddy. I could see through the living-room into the dining-room, which was likewise empty. The mother explained that these rooms have been closed off for the winter months, since it is quite expensive to heat them and the family doesn't actually need them. She opened the door and led me into the hall-way in which Jerry's crib is kept, and from there we proceeded to the kitchen.

'The kitchen is bright, cheery and well equipped. It contains a large oil stove which heats the entire back part of the house. I saw a handsome new electric refrigerator which the family has not had for long. In the middle of the kitchen is a fairly large dining-room table covered with a plastic cloth, and around it were a number of comfortable chairs. The cabinets and the sink are of fairly late design. There is an additional closet, probably used for mops or some such thing, which is concealed by white cotton drapes trimmed with red. Almost everything in the kitchen is white with red trimming.

'The parents' bedroom looked attractive. It contained a new modern bedroom suite; the colour scheme in this bedroom is dark rose and light-brown. The other bedroom, which is used by Freddy,

[1]In this section of the United States, the paradoxical situation is that families who cannot afford the rent for a simple house or apartment can (and are almost compelled to) buy a house. Mortgages are arranged in such a way that the monthly instalments toward payment of the debt are less than rent would have been. On such long-range financing the drawback is that interest considerably adds to the debt, and that by the time the family own the house outright, it may be so old as to be of low value and of a size no longer suitable to a family that has doubled or tripled in the meantime.

is furnished a little shabbily, and apparently is used as a living-room as well as sleeping-quarters for Freddy. It contained a well-used studio couch, several old chairs, a small table or cabinet and boxes of Freddy's toys. Apparently this room does not have a closet, because Freddy's clothing was hanging from a number of brackets in the hall-way. In the kitchen doorway hung Jerry's jumper.[1] All of the rooms appeared very clean and orderly.'

The mother's personality will reveal itself, we think, as the reader learns how she behaved with her baby, how she responded to us, and how she expressed her thoughts and feelings, not only about the baby and his care, but about her values, interests, hopes and fears. We shall introduce her, therefore, only by a description of her appearance and manner as these impressed us after our first contact with her (drawn from our original records). This will be followed by a brief résumé of her past history.

'The mother is an attractive though not pretty woman whom I would judge to be in her middle twenties. She is of medium height, slender, and her figure is not well developed. Her face appears actually thin; I believe this is emphasized by a long nose. Her dark, soft, fluffy hair appeared rather dishevelled, and I think this was because it was arranged in small ringlets which had been blown by the wind on the way to the Centre. It is shoulder-length and this plus a curly, short, high bang, again tends to emphasize the length and the thinness of her face. Her mouth is rather narrow and when she smiles she exposes rather long teeth which are not altogether even. Her brows, which were conservatively plucked, do not extend as far either laterally or medially as is usual. She was wearing bright lipstick but little other make-up. She has rather beautiful soft blue eyes. Her eyes and her face, which is mobile, quietly tend to reflect various feeling states with the result that at times she momentarily appeared almost beautiful. Her movements tended to be moderately slow, and her voice was so quiet that at times it was difficult to hear her.

'She wore a brown and white seersucker dress that was certainly not of this year's style, and that showed evidence of a good deal of washing, but which was fresh and neat-looking. It had short sleeves and a peplum, and tied in the front at the opening of the

---

[1] A jumper or jumper-swing is a little canvas seat on a metal frame suspended on chains which are fastened to hooks in a doorway or archway. Usually, as in this home, the seat hangs low enough so that the baby's feet can touch the ground. The baby sits securely as the canvas surrounds the trunk. It is possible for him to stand thus, to kick the floor and cause the seat to swing, or to be pushed so that the swing moves in a wider arc.

rather high round neckline. Her shoes were black suède and open; I believe low-heeled. She wore cameo earrings which hardly showed beneath the halo of hair, and on one hand her wedding ring with a second ring which had a small red stone, on the other a silver band with an embossed design. Her nails were enamelled pink.'

The mother was born and reared in one of the beautiful north-western states of America where she lived with her family until she married at the age of nineteen. They were a fairly large family who were close to one another emotionally and in their interests, even after the children had grown to be young adults. The entire family was musically inclined and Jerry's grandmother (maternal) had professional training as a pianist. Each family member played an instrument or sang; the mother was interested enough to obtain some voice training during her high school years. In addition the family as a whole customarily went fishing, picnicking and the like. The mother's parents and one sibling had died within three years of the time we spoke with her, and she still seemed to feel an acute sense of loss and a sort of loneliness in response to the break-up of this family unit.

The mother met the father when he was stationed at a military base near her home. He was transferred to the West Coast after they had known each other for only two weeks. When he received his orders for service overseas (this was during the war), he proposed by telephone and she accepted. When she set out on her thousand-mile journey to marry a man she hardly knew, it was also her first separation from home. They had a few weeks together before he left, and the mother worked in several places during the years of separation, not returning home except to visit. Prior to her marriage she had worked in a book-shop and especially enjoyed it for she was allowed to take home the books she wished to read. Her jobs after marriage were varied, including selling in stores and clerking in a ship-yard. Shortly after the father's discharge they moved to the city where her husband grew up and where our study was done. The mother was a Catholic, but did not seem troubled by the fact that the father was not. She saw to it that the children were baptized properly, and considered it 'my duty and obligation' to provide instruction for them in the Catholic faith. She gave us to understand that in her opinion any religion is all right 'as long as you have one'. The moderation of her views is also apparent from the fact that she planned for the children to attend public school (not parochial) because she believed that it provides richer experience, and that one can be a good Catholic without attending parochial school.

About the father we knew very much less. He impressed the observers as moderately tall, nice-looking. Some of us regarded him as somewhat effeminate in appearance, others did not share this impression. Certainly, when the whole family visited briefly at our offices, he behaved in a very maternal fashion with Freddy, looking after him and entertaining him so that the mother might be free to chat with us.

The father had lived in this community all his life, with the exception of the time spent in military service. His mother and two married brothers lived in our town as well, and the various branches of the family visited with one another a good deal. It seemed to the mother that the members of her husband's family were not especially close to one another and had few mutual interests. The father was raised as a member of one of the Protestant churches; again it seemed to the mother that the father was scarcely a religious person although he had remained a member of his church. He had no objection to having his children reared as Catholics. He completed high school and received intensive special training with a local railroad company as a machinist. He worked for this company still and it is probable that, like many men in our town, which happens to be a railroad centre, he more or less expected to work for them all his life. As to his personality, the mother described him as an active sort of person who is up and doing something all the time. He was, she thought, quick-tempered, but apparently his anger was a thing of the moment. She held him to be a very dependable person who would force himself to go to work even when he felt ill. It may seem as if the mother's description of the father was rather a critical and distant one. Actually, this was hardly the case. While this mother was not a person given to the verbal expression of personal feelings (whether tender or otherwise), she conveyed a sense of warmth and at-one-ness with the father indirectly. For instance, in describing to us how toilet-training had been managed with Freddy, or how they coped with the fact that relatives were critical of her second pregnancy, the mother spoke of how 'we decided' in such a manner as to convey that the parents really shared interest and responsibility for details of child care and for larger decisions as well. She also quoted conversations between herself and the father which showed that he was receptive toward her interests and attitudes even when he did not share them, and that she was comfortable in expressing to him things which might be taken as criticisms of his way of life or his family members.

Freddy was an exceptionally engaging little boy. He had sandy hair, very fair skin, and large blue eyes. He tended to move about rapidly, enjoyed climbing, running, riding his tricycle, etc.; the mother thought him the more active of her two sons. Yet he also enjoyed books and imaginative play rather more than do most two-and-a-half-year-olds. The mother thought that with respect to temperament Freddy resembled his father more than herself, being curious, excitable, quick to anger and quick to change over to a happy mood again. From his response to the radio and to her singing, she felt it likely that he possessed musical talent, and hoped that he could have music lessons later on. The parents also were proud of what seemed to them his mechanical ability. The father spent a good deal of time (evenings and Sundays) with Freddy, and the latter 'worked' with his father, apparently demonstrating interest and perhaps skill, in the use of tools. The mother's diary record of his development indicated that Freddy had developed rather rapidly, especially with respect to bodily skills. He had his second tooth at three and a half months, said 'mamma' at six months and several simple words at eleven months. He fed himself by hand at thirteen months, and could use a spoon adequately at thirteen and a half months. At one year he lifted his legs to get his feet into his trousers, at thirteen months he combed his hair, and he blew his nose and tried to put on his own shoes at fourteen months.

When we knew him, Freddy was an expressive youngster; he spoke a great deal and showed no shyness at all. He talked so rapidly and indistinctly that the mother often had to interpret his meaning to the observer. We were interested to note that he thoroughly enjoyed make-believe. He was seen to carry out quite elaborate fantasy games involving a car accident and the attendant rescue activities, and delightedly 'servicing' the observer with imaginary water, etc., so she might wash her hands. The mother clearly encouraged imaginative play and entered it actively on several occasions. According to her, Freddy had at first ignored the baby, showing no open resentment and no positive interest. More recently, since Jerry had been interested in toys and shared more actively in family life, Freddy had spent quite a bit of time with the baby. From the anecdotes the mother told, we received the impression that Freddy's interest in Jerry was often a friendly and playful one, but that he also tended to become too rough, as when he would swing the baby so high that the latter cried, or patted his head rather too hard. He jealously guarded his toys, but would also give the baby some of his when in a generous mood. The parents had seen to it that Freddy received as much attention after the baby was born as he had before. We saw the mother uphold Freddy's right to take his toy away from Jerry, although she first asked if he would not lend it to the baby. To the observer she explained having read that 'if you make the older one give his things to the baby it only makes his jealousy worse'.

The star performer was Jerry himself, and the aim of this writing is to convey a sense of what he was like. Physically he was 'the spittin' image' of his older brother. Fair, blue-eyed, blond with a reddish glint to his hair, expressive, mobile and active. His mother thought him of a more quiet disposition than the brother, more like herself and less like the father. 'He has a temper but he doesn't show it so often'.

PREGNANCY AND DELIVERY

The mother described her pregnancy as having been an exceptionally smooth one. Her stomach felt uneasy a time or two but otherwise she felt very well. Her mood was no different from what it ordinarily was; she did not experience the irritability or mood-swings which she had observed in some of the pregnant women she knew.

The delivery was at term and also free from complications. She began to feel light pains at 7.30 in the morning. They became severe only by 6 or 6.30 the same evening. She went to the hospital at 6 p.m., and at first the doctors thought the baby would not be born until the following morning. However, by 8 p.m. the 'water broke', and the baby arrived shortly before midnight. During the evening the mother was given shots.[1] During the delivery itself ether was administered and the mother remembered 'going under' and 'waking up' again several times. Toward the end, and before the baby was actually born, she received enough anaesthetic to become completely unconscious and did not waken until three hours after the baby's birth. Quite vividly the mother described how she awoke in a darkened hallway (the hospital was crowded and it was some hours until a bed could be made free), and saw nothing but the large electric wall clock. 'I thought I was in the next world'. She felt her abdomen to see if the baby had been born. A nurse soon came and gave her ice which relieved the nausea, and also told her about the baby and the fact that the father had been there earlier. It was at this time the mother learned that she had another boy. Without embarrassment she told us that she had hoped for a girl, as had the father. However, from the moment after she first saw the baby (the next morning when he was ten hours old), she never thought about it again and felt content to have a boy. To her relief the father also assured her that he did not mind, 'as long as it is healthy and has ten fingers and ten toes we'll keep it', he told her jokingly.

Following the delivery the mother lost a good deal of hair (this had also been true after Freddy's birth). She was convinced that this, as well as some trouble with her teeth, was related to her pregnancies, although she had been told that this was 'just a woman's notion'.

Mother and baby remained in the hospital for five and a half days after his birth. Her recovery was smooth, she sat up the second day,

[1]Sedation by means of injections are routinely given to women in labour in this and the majority of American hospitals. They induce drowsiness but not sleep, so the mother can still co-operate with instructions, but her awareness of pain (and of everything else) is dulled.

left the bed briefly on the third, and began to walk about more freely on the fourth day. During this time Freddy spent his days in the home of his paternal grandmother, but slept at home with his father. This arrangement continued for a few days after the mother's return from the hospital.

The baby was declared to be altogether healthy and normal at birth. His birth-weight was 7 lb. 2 oz. The mother did not attempt to breast-feed him at all because she had had 'bad luck' with Freddy (her lactation was inadequate). He received a synthetic milk formula[1] on a regular four-hour schedule running through the twenty-four-hour period. The mother fed him twice daily, the other times he was fed in the nursery (this also is hospital routine). He had diarrhoea in the hospital. It was later thought that he could not tolerate the formula because the trouble disappeared as soon as another preparation was used. At any rate he lost some weight, so that on his sixth day, upon discharge from the hospital, he weighed 6 lb. 14 oz. This was not lasting, however, for when next he was weighed at nine weeks he weighed over 10 lb., which was considered a good gain in relation to his birth-weight.

JERRY'S DEVELOPMENT UP TO THE AGE OF SEVEN MONTHS

Physical growth and health

All in all Jerry was a very healthy baby. As already mentioned, he had diarrhoea upon return from the hospital, which persisted until he was between three and four weeks old. His stools were liquid and almost every diaper was stained. His sleep was irregular and at times disturbed during these weeks, and the mother thought that he often had gas on his stomach and cried from this cause. Being held upright and patted until he burped was often effective in getting him back to sleep, as was an extra feeding. A medicine was prescribed (mother no longer remembered its name) and seemed to help him. His skin in the region of the buttocks was sore and irritated. However, he ate well, slept a good amount, and while not really well, he apparently was not really sick either, at that time. The mother did not consider having a doctor see him as she felt advice received by telephone was adequate.

---

[1]A great many preparations for baby formulae crowd the American market. Many are packaged in powdered form and need only to be mixed with sterile water. They usually contain vitamins and some other substances in addition to the equivalent of the nutritive components of natural milk. Those able to afford the slightly higher price often prefer this to the work involved in preparing formula. For the same reason, hospitals often use such 'packaged' milk.

His recovery was attributed to the combined effects of the medication and the change in formula (evaporated milk).

Since that time, age four weeks, no illness had occurred. With the first introduction to vegetables (at twelve weeks) and to meat (at twenty-two weeks) there was both times a slight recurrence of the diarrhoea, which lasted less than twenty-four hours each time. Twice he had a minor cold, once when barely over six months old and once just as he became seven months. There was no fever, no real diarrhoea, but for a few days his stools were somewhat loose and the number of bowel movements per day increased to about seven. This was possibly due to the fact that the mother applied a home remedy (castor oil, ¼ teaspoon) which has a laxative effect.

Jerry was seen by a doctor on his sixth day, upon discharge from the hospital; at nine weeks; and from then on once a month at the local Public Health Department Well Baby Clinic.[1] Always he was pronounced a healthy baby. Jerry was thus spared many of the common minor ailments of infancy. He had no skin-rashes, no 'colic', he did not spit up or vomit (except once when given pure pork meat at five months) and had no inexplicable crying spells.

Feeding History

It will be remembered that Jerry was never breast-fed, and that in the hospital he received a formula prepared from a synthetic product. Probably for economic reasons, though the mother did not say so, he was changed to a formula prepared with evaporated milk.[2] To begin with the proportion was 6 oz. of evaporated milk to 10 oz. of water. No sugar was added because of his tendency to have loose stools. Gradually the proportion was changed so that, some time before we met him, the proportions of canned milk and water were equal, i.e. he was receiving the equivalent of natural undiluted cow's milk.

Cereal was given first at six weeks of age, to this was added canned

[1]The Well Baby Clinics are maintained by government personnel, they are open to any member of the community and restrict themselves to the paediatric supervision of healthy children. The doctor examines the baby, he is weighed, and the mother receives advice concerning his diet and other routine aspects of his care. The inoculations required by law are administered free of charge. In the case of inexperienced or overburdened mothers, public health nurses may also visit the home and help the mother in carrying out the doctor's recommendations.

[2]American manufacturers produce small cans of evaporated milk of a size convenient for formula preparation. The strength is standardized to be exactly twice that of cow's milk. Thus doctors usually instruct mothers about the baby's formula in terms of: so much water mixed with the contents of one can. The evaporated milk is considered safer, and it certainly is cheaper than fresh pasteurized milk.

strained fruit at twelve weeks, and canned strained vegetables at about fifteen weeks.[1] At twenty-two weeks meat was recommended (also canned and strained) but he did not respond well to pork, which happened to be the only pure meat the neighbourhood store had available. The mother began to give him meat and vegetable mixtures and, as they agreed with him, she did not try other meats. Some time after age five and a half months, egg yolk, pudding, plain vanilla cookies and some bland fresh fruits such as bananas were added to his diet. We think it important to mention that the mother did not offer orange juice for some time after the first two or three attempts because it seemed to her that he did not like the sour taste. Similarly, hard boiled egg was recommended but Jerry did not like it, spat it out and would not swallow it. Apparently it did not even occur to his mother to 'train' him to accept the disliked food as many other mothers might have done, but she experimented with various consistencies until she found he liked the egg, provided it was soft boiled. She also respected other food dislikes: for instance he 'made faces' when given peas, and after she had exhausted her supply the mother did not offer them again.

The mother made no special effort to maintain a feeding schedule, but found that for the most part Jerry became hungry at regular intervals. The first few weeks he still received a 2 a.m. bottle, but then no longer accepted food at that hour though he sometimes awakened. In order to help him sleep through the night the mother gave him his 'big meal' (fruits and vegetables) at 10 p.m. for a while, with his last bottle. (As far as we can reconstruct, this was customary for him between approximately four and a half and six and a half months.) At age six and a half months, he began to have his supper with the whole family, in his high-chair[2], but at the table with the others, at about 6 o'clock in the evening. He was then given a bedtime bottle between

[1]American mothers are fortunate in that an almost infinite variety of 'baby foods' is available in small-sized cans. Oatmeal, barley and similar cereals, as well as every kind of fruit, vegetable and meat (and mixtures of these) are available in strained form for infants, and chopped form for children old enough to begin chewing their food. This is not only an enormous saving in time, but the cost is below what it would be if the raw materials had to be bought and prepared at home.

[2]The high-chair is almost a universal piece of equipment for babies in American homes. It is a wooden stool-like structure with a seat at a height of the average kitchen table. The baby sits completely enclosed; in front is a tray at a height convenient for him to put his arms on. The sides and back are enclosed by bars or boards. Unless he were to slide downwards (which is difficult to do) the baby is thus secure at a height convenient to adults. Most babies enjoy the high-chair, perhaps because it affords a better view of the environs than most other spots where they are apt to be put down.

8 and 8.30 p.m. Since then he has not required food between 8 p.m. and 7 to 8 a.m.

All his life Jerry has been allowed to go to sleep over his bottle, always at night time and usually for day-time naps as well. When tiny, the mother held him in her arms for feedings. She then found (we do not know just when), that during the day he ate better and fell asleep more readily if he was in the crib and the bottle propped up beside his head. He was held at night until night feedings ceased altogether.

The mother said that Jerry has always been eager for his food and that it is typical for him to eat very rapidly. This is true both for bottle and spoon feedings. Except on rare occasions Jerry has received his food only from the mother. However, when left at the grandmother's house at times, he readily accepted food from her as well. The father has occasionally given him his bottle when the mother was out, but never attempted a spoon feeding.

It was our impression that the mother had a wholesome positive yet casual attitude toward feedings. She seemed to take for granted that food is something to be enjoyed, and avoided foods the baby disliked. Yet she made no fuss, did not watch just how much he consumed but stopped when he seemed to have had enough. Sometimes she warmed his food and other times she gave it at room temperature; and she stopped sterilizing the water and the bottle earlier than the doctor recommended. She explained that neighbours' children of like age were getting along fine though their mothers did not sterilize any more, so she felt it was safe to do likewise.

Development and Life Situation

When mother and baby returned from the hospital the household was, of course, somewhat disrupted. The mother was still weak, and the father did most of the necessary housework when he returned home from work in the evening. Jerry slept in a small crib in his parents' bedroom. Except for being looked at by visiting relatives, his only human contact was with his mother who fed him, held him when he seemed restless, clothed him and bathed him. The latter was done with unusual gentleness. The mother held the baby in her arms and, exposing only portions of his body at a time, sponged and immediately dried him. A little later she still held him but began to dip his legs and other parts of the body into a small pan to rinse him, but did not yet lower him into the basin. Some time later she began letting him sit in the small pan, which was still the method used at seven months. By that time the mother thought he would 'soon' be old enough to be comfortable in a larger pan or tub.

After the family resumed its normal style of living, the baby was fairly remote from the hustle and bustle. The bedroom where his crib stood was barely used during the day, his brother more or less ignored him, and neither parent believed that young babies should be played with very actively. After recovery from diarrhoea he adopted a regular pattern of eating and sleeping. While taking care of him, the mother spoke and sang to him, he was brought into the living-room occasionally, the father might talk to him, pat him or tickle him playfully for a while in the evening, but he was not rocked, or bounced and tossed, or taken out much. On fine days he slept out of doors at times, and every once in a while he was deposited with his grandmother for an evening while the parents went out. In his mother's arms he was taken on car rides or to the store on occasion, and once a month he was taken to the Well Baby Clinic.

The mother wrote down some of his developmental gains during this early period, enough to show that his physical growth and awareness of things increased in about the normal way. At six weeks he smiled responsively, at seven and a half weeks he would smile at the sound of the mother's voice even if he could not see her. At two months he turned his head in the direction of whoever happened to be speaking near by, and at three month he held his head steadily erect in the sitting position.

At about three months he became a more active participant in family life and gradually expanded the range and variety of his experience. He was transferred to a larger crib which stood in the hallway communicating with the family's daytime living space. The mother felt that Jerry enjoyed this new arrangement, and spent much time simply watching what went on about him. Toys were always near, first his own and then his brother's as well. A good proportion of his earliest contacts with Freddy appear to have consisted of the latter's giving the baby toys and taking them from his hands. The parents felt that they did not need to teach him how to use toys (as they had with Freddy) for he would learn enough just watching his brother. We received the impression, however, that while the mother did not intentionally teach him, she was more aware of his need for playthings, and provided more opportunity for object-exploration, than many mothers might, i.e., she made a rattle for him by stringing together some old piano keys, and she was able to tell us which colours he seemed to prefer for his toys.

While he continued to spend a good deal of waking time in the crib, there was an increasing number of other possible spots for him in the house. Some time between the ages of four and five and a half months he began to use the jumper-swing and the high-chair. He might be on his parents' bed, on the divan or a big chair for a time, he was taken car-riding more often, and week-end visits to relatives were the rule. He was kept off the floor carefully, because the mother thought it draughty (which it was), and for this reason a play-pen was not used.

The range of his social contacts also increased. Not only did he interact more with his father and brother than before, but he was included in the situation when visitors came, which occurred often. The mother said that he cried very seldom, except when hungry or in other discomfort, as for instance, when his diapers were soiled, or he lost his balance and fell, or when he dropped a toy and could not recover it. In her opinion, a baby who cries just from 'temper' and not from real discomfort should not be comforted at once but rather left to cry it out. Emphasizing that with Jerry this occurred but seldom, she explained that she has known children who were spoiled in this manner, and thinks that they were 'backward' in their development. In the same context she also said that those allowed to find their own way out of minor difficulties are 'more independent'. Observation of this mother with her children led us to think that the mother did not fully describe her own attitude. We did see her watch the baby fuss or cry without doing something about it. However, much more typically she forestalled the occurrence of distress. When the baby began to squirm restlessly, or disregard his toys, or vocalize a bit plaintively, she tended almost automatically to change his position, offer him a different toy, or speculate whether he might be getting hungry or sleepy.

Under these circumstances Jerry continued to grow, as partially reflected in the mother's diary notes. At three and a half months he watched the movement of his hands and laughed out loud. At four months he reached for and held a toy, and at five months he turned to look after a toy that had fallen from his hands. At five and a half months he rolled from his back on to his stomach, and by six months he gave unmistakable signs of distinguishing between familiar persons and strangers.

JERRY AND HIS WORLD AT 7 MONTHS

Over-all Characteristics

As three observers watched Jerry through one afternoon of his life, saw him respond to sights and sounds, to movement and touch, to his mother and to toys, there formed in their minds a distinct impression of Jerry as a person. This 'over-all impression' was put in writing by each one, before a detailed analysis of his observed behaviour had been made. Impressionistic formulations of this sort typically overstress some, and omit other aspects, but since they also communicate a more unified perception, we shall introduce Jerry through some of these descriptions.

'The baby is a very active, unusually energetic, sturdy-appearing, handsome child. He has a nicely rounded head, ears a little more prominent than usual, his facial features are rather coarse though handsome, his shoulders are broad and his hands and feet are large. He has a small amount of straight yellowish brown hair with a reddish cast to it. He has the thin pinkish white skin frequently seen in redheads. At times his cheeks were very rosy. There was some dried saliva or mucus about his mouth and nose but apart from this he appeared clean. He has very light pale brows and lashes and his eyes are light, rather pale blue.

'In the perceptual sphere he seems somehow less sensitive than many children we see. He looked about with interest and curiosity, gazing at people and things directly and often letting his mouth hang open a little. Yet as a rule his regard is not sustained for any length of time and I did not get the impression that visual stimuli were especially pleasing nor at all distressing to him. When awake, he often attended to sounds in the room but again tended to lose interest in them quickly. He was not awakened by loud, sudden, sharp noises, though he occasionally appeared to react to them as he slept. He appeared to be a child with a good deal of drive who derives considerable pleasure from active movement and manipulation of objects, and who is unable to behave, or not interested in behaving, as the passive receptor of environmental stimulation. He showed few signs of receptively savouring experiences or stimuli offered by the environment. Rather he tends to pay minimal attention to these, to turn from them quickly and return to his own pleasurable activity. I recall his taking time out to attend to the external environment only when the mother stimulated him in a particular way, which consisted of her sitting quietly a foot or two away from him and talking to him very softly yet with her face reflecting some excitement and eagerness. At such times Jerry remained comparatively still, he regarded the mother for what was for him a prolonged period of time and puffed softly and excitedly. With the investigators he was not at all socially responsive; he seemed neither frightened of them nor particularly desirous of contact with them.

'When shown toys he responded immediately, reaching vigorously for them and giving up whatever he already had. It seemed to me that once he had the toy he often used it as an extension of his own body rather than as something external to himself. It was

142

my impression that comparatively strong responses of pleasure and displeasure were to be seen in the tactile and kinaesthetic areas. When "A" touched his skin in testing tissue resistance he became unusually still; when I touched his abdomen he tried to push my hands away and his facial expression reflected some displeasure, I thought. As already stated, he appeared to enjoy active movement very much, and when restrained, as in being dressed, he showed his displeasure by resisting and fussing. One always knew what he wanted or did not want. As a rule, it was clear that he was either in a fairly good or bad mood; there were seldom any in-between states. With fatigue or frustration he yelled at once. There were exceptionally few indications of nuances of feelings.

'While in most respects his behaviour is compatible with average or high average standards for his age, yet, comparing him with the superior twenty-eight and thirty-two-week-old infants we have seen, he appeared not at all bright, and also his behaviour seemed stereotyped and lacking in variability. A good deal of Jerry's activity consisted in rolling, slapping, patting, waving, shaking, banging, scratching, etc. Also he not infrequently played rather gently with his own body.

'In respect to language development Jerry is actually retarded. I believe that a few polysyllabic vowel sounds were heard, as is to be expected at twenty-eight week age-level, but these were not at all distinct. As a rule he vocalized vigorously and the vocalizations were lacking in variability as was the rest of his behaviour. Also I thought that they failed to reflect nuances in feeling just as did his facial expressions and movements. He was dressed in diaper, vest, red and white striped T-shirt, well-worn grey corduroy overalls, white shoes, sweater and knitted cap.'

Another observer saw Jerry as follows:

'Jerry is a large, muscular, fair-skinned, long boy with a small quantity of red blondish hair and very large round blue eyes. He is decidedly masculine in appearance in spite of the fact that his genital organs seem relatively small. His skin was smooth and free from blemishes except for a bruise on the temple which the mother told us he sustained when he took a hard fall recently. Respirations seemed no longer abdominal in type and hence could not be observed. They were inaudible except for brief periods of time when he engaged in a sort of puffing excited breathing which seemed more like a means of expressing pleasurable excitement than an involuntary characteristic of the respiratory system. He flushed very rarely and then moderately; twice it was observed when he was crying loudly and once or twice just prior to a deep burp. His

143

movements were vigorous, moderately rapid and quite extensive. Neuro-muscular strength would seem to be excellent in that he requires very little support when standing, propels himself about when in the crib and showed excellent head support. His postures and movements were of high average or slightly accelerated calibre in comparison to norms for his age. When picking up and regarding toys, at least in the sitting position as during the psychological test, the right eye frequently and briefly showed an internal strabismus.

'All of his responses appeared to be immediate, vigorous, robust and active rather than discriminative, observant or sensitively differentiated. He showed almost no observable reaction to contact with unfamiliar people and strange surroundings. In fact, I was struck with the fact that his play with one of the toys, the bead string, very early in the experiment, was identical with his play with the same object toward the very end of the experiment. Beyond this, his very active play with toys was stereotyped in that he did the same things with all toys as much as possible, paying very little attention to the different characteristics of the objects he handled. Whether it was the bead string, rattles, the rubber toy, blocks or the bell, all of them would be swung about, banged, transferred, lifted to the mouth for brief periods of time, and sometimes dropped deliberately. He not only frequently brought objects to the mouth, where he tended to champ and chew on them rather than to lick them, but would also occasionally bring his mouth to objects. Intense or prolonged mouthing was not observed and he sucked his finger only once while fussing.

'He is the only infant in the research group so far whom I have observed to engage in what I thought was deliberate and purposive genital play. This occurred as the mother was changing his diaper and did not persist for long. His vocalizations, which came forth readily and often, were loud, and seemed less well differentiated to me than is the case with most children of like age. They consisted of not very clear single vowel sounds, mixed vowel sounds which were occasionally multi-syllabic, and squeals. His facial expression and social responsiveness also were vigorous rather than sensitive. He regarded his mother as well as the investigators with fascination and interest quite frequently, but never for long. As already mentioned, he did not show shrinking or apprehensiveness or anything like anxiety. He would either regard a person or an object open-mouthed and with wide open eyes as if very alertly interested, or sometimes grin broadly. There were no fleeting smiles and he was not heard to chuckle or laugh.

'His relative lack of sensitivity also seemed to be reflected in his

144

enjoyment of noises of such intensity as are at least mildly irritating to most other infants. He would bang the bell or other hard objects on the metal top of the table as forcefully as it was possible to do, and seemed to enjoy the better, the louder the resulting sound, without blinking or any other sign of responding to the harshness of the stimulus. From the fact that he showed minimal disturbance, and usually none, when he fell quite forcefully, especially from the sitting position, one would judge that he is not especially sensitive to pain either. I was not able to observe any response to the photographic illumination, although I was not in a position to see him when the lights first went on. This baby never left any doubt as to his likes and dislikes in a given situation. He either withdrew from something, making clearly objecting and irritated noises, or screaming loudly; or else he would forcefully and with signs of pleasure approach objects and situations.'

The third observer agreed with most of what has already been said, but emphasized the purposiveness of Jerry's behaviour in a somewhat different form:

'The most striking thing about his general behaviour was the intensity of his interest in objects. When "B"[1], for instance, laid the hoop on the table, he gave what was almost a sob at the sight of it and lunged forward toward it across the table with his whole body and reached it almost immediately. When I tried to rate his handgrip he had a string of beads over one hand. When I slipped the chain of beads off, which was easy to do, he made searching movements with the hand from which the beads were removed and showed no interest in grasping with the other hand until they had been replaced. When "B" removed the cup and spoon during the test he showed behaviour which I described as a small tantrum, and when the cup later reappeared there was heavy breathing, almost 'panting' or 'wheezing' at the sight of it. It took longer in general for him to accept the disappearance of an object that he was interested in, than other babies I have so far observed.

'He showed definite evidence of living beyond the immediate situation both in his behaviour when objects disappeared and again in his behaviour when the bottle was presented. In that case he had been crying vigorously but became quiet at the sight of a bottle well before it was placed in direct relationship to his mouth.

'He also showed specific object preferences, the shiny cup and spoon being special favourites. His mother told that he liked strong

[1]Editor's note: 'A' and 'B' have been substituted for the names of the members of the research team involved.

145

colours, red and also black and white, more than pastel shades. In his motor play with objects he found satisfaction in a rather discriminative kind of banging. For instance, he banged one test object directly on the taped corner of the little metal table, then moved around so as to bang it on the corner of the little wooden table beside his mother's chair. This activity showed both exactness of co-ordination and a high degree of articulation of his visual environment which made these corners stand out as something special which it was both possible and 'fun' to treat in a special way.

'All in all, he was an energetic, purposeful baby whose goal behaviour was more highly motivated than that of many babies and who more frequently suffered frustration in the midst of a situation such as ours. His mother spoke of his "temper" in these situations. However, he showed rather quick recovery from these disturbances and soon found something else to interest him when one goal was interfered with. He had not been in the office long before he began to be fussy, and his mother finally decided that he was hungry although it was not yet time for him to eat. I had the impression from this and from the way in which he later settled down for a nap that, although the situation was a fairly strenuous one for him, he showed good ability to handle himself in it. When we finally awakened him to finish our observations he came to himself gradually and seemed fresh and happy'.

The above statements are, of course, condensed inferences from the observation of Jerry as he responded to a multitude of situations. Traits such as 'vigour' or 'selectiveness' or 'alertness' have no meaning except as they come to expression in the continuity of concrete specific situations which constitute his existence. Their significance can be understood only in the context of the particular range of situations which were available to Jerry for him to react to. It would be our view that his individuality as a person, and even his emotional health, are defined by the characteristics of his environment almost as much as by the characteristics which he as an organism brought to it. In the sections to follow we shall make no attempt to separate the two, though once his mode of functioning has been described, a more systematic statement may be profitable.

Jerry and His World of Things

At seven months of age a child has reached the point where he is aware of the difference between objects and persons. While it is true that he does not understand the nature and purpose of things as he will a few years later, and while he may occasionally respond to his

146

mother's hand or to his own foot much as one would to a thing, he nevertheless has expectations in relation to objects which are quite different from those he manifests in relation to people. Correspondingly, the kinds of activity that occur in interaction with things are widely different from those arising from interaction with persons. This is so not only because people behave differently than do things, but also because of the child's awareness of this difference. Needless to say, such awareness need not be intellectual comprehension.

The following examples are more or less representative of hundreds of others contained in our observational records of this child's behaviour.

During the afternoon he spent with us, Jerry maintained an active relationship with one or several objects almost continuously, except while sleeping.[1] It would be difficult to say to what extent this was a function of the fact that his mother continually offered toys, and to what extent he chose to direct his attention to objects. The most prolonged exposure to a variety of objects occurred during the psychological test which largely consists of presenting a variety of objects. The following incidents are chosen more or less at random from the description of his test behaviour.

' "B" presented a cube. The baby immediately picked it up. "B" presented a second cube. The baby banged them against one another and on the table. When the third cube was held in front of him, he touched it with the cube that he was already holding, and approached it with his mouth. Mass of cubes: the baby picked up two cubes, one in each hand, and hit and pushed the other cubes with them. He was completely preoccupied with his play, appeared rather relaxed. He gave the impression of a person who is happily busy. All of his energy which formerly had gone into moving about on the mother's lap, reaching for the side of the chair, etc., now seemed to go into play with the toys. He hit the table with the cubes. He appeared able to hold the cube easily with three fingers. The cup was offered while he still had two cubes. He immediately hit the cup with one cube, then let go of one cube in favour of picking up the cup. Now he held a cube in one hand and a cup in the other. He banged the cup vigorously against the table.

'Bell: the infant reached for it immediately; I did not see how he picked it up. He transferred it adeptly. He banged the table with it,

[1]This is not always the case in the same situation; i.e., while the world of objects surrounds all children most of the time, many ignore them for periods of time or expend but little energy in their exploration. Jerry differed from many of the thirty-two-week-olds whom we studied in the same manner by his intense reactivity to the things about him.

repeatedly rang it and at such times his mouth fell open a little and his face was very sober, he banged it against the table again. Squeaky doll: characteristically the baby reached for a toy the very instant he saw it and easily gave up the toy he already had in its favour. He immediately brought the doll to his mouth, but didn't do much but hold it in the mouth briefly. He shook it. He slapped the table top with it. He seemed completely preoccupied in this play. Pellet in bottle: the baby paid no attention when the pellet fell out of the bottle. He was interested only in the bottle which he banged against the table.

' "B" now removes the other objects and puts the hoop with the string attached on the table. The baby practically cries with eagerness as he sees it and reaches for it. In reaching for the hoop with his hand, he gets his arm on the string and moves the string with the arm in such a way that he is just able to finger the hoop. His attention all the time was on the hoop and not at all on the string'.

The psychological test report summed up Jerry's behaviour in relation to test objects as follows:

'Throughout the test Jerry tended to respond to the objects offered, in a most vigorous manner. His responses followed immediately upon perception of the stimulus, and when there was any delay either in presentation or in his performing the necessary motions in order to obtain the object he gave every sign of impatience. That is, his facial expression would reflect distress and something like anger, his movements would become jerky, and not infrequently he turned away from the task unhappily. In view of this extremely vigorous responsiveness it is not surprising that as testing proceeded muscular tension manifestations became rather conspicuous. While normally responsive socially, on other occasions Jerry became so absorbed with and excited over the test objects that he made practically no social responses to the examiner in the course of testing'.

Whether on his mother's lap, in the crib, or on the floor, Jerry did not wait for objects to be brought toward him, nor did he lose interest when they disappeared (unless an attractive substitute was immediately available).

'Again the mother brought him to a standing position on her lap. He was holding two toys. Her hands were at his waist. He bent down as far as he could go toward her knees. He dropped a toy, bent down still further and appeared about to go after it with his whole body. He kept his gaze fixed on it.'

'The baby gave up his toys and played with the suitcase. He patted it, slapped it, fingered it, and two or three times he brought his mouth to the plastic handle of the case. He would open his mouth as he brought it toward the handle, contact the handle briefly with open mouth, then draw his head away at once.

'He manipulated the diaper on which his bottle had been propped, in one or both hands. The mother took the diaper from him, giving him the toy rubber duck in its place. He accepted the duck and did not seem to mind that the diaper was taken from him. He played with the duck and also with his own feet, which he grasped.'

Play with toys, in his case, was frequently combined with other activities. Whether he was feeding or being dressed, weighed, bathed or otherwise manipulated, he seldom lost an opportunity to grasp things, wave them, bang them, bring them to the mouth, drop them and retrieve them. The scene below occurred towards the end of a bottle-feeding. He had been drinking with the bottle propped on some folded diapers by the side of the head. He had lost the nipple from his mouth without protesting, and the mother did not seem to be certain whether or not he was still hungry.

'The mother then placed the bottle in his hands and he grasped it. There followed a fascinating and somewhat amusing scene which all of us, including the mother, watched with absorption, so that for a minute or two there was no conversation whatsoever. The baby held and manipulated and regarded the bottle in an excited manner. He would wave it about using both hands, change his hold upon it, sometimes hold the glass part with one hand and manipulate, bend and twist the nipple with his other hand. The longer he played with it the more excited he seemed to become. The excitement manifested itself in an exaggerated kind of respiratory noise which one might describe as "puffing". He thus breathed rapidly and loudly. I was under the impression that this was an almost deliberate playful thing rather than an accidental by-product of excitement. Since he moved the bottle about very rapidly it was difficult to be sure of this, but I was not under the impression that the baby was trying to get the nipple into his mouth, rather he seemed to be just playing with the bottle.

'I thought it interesting that the mother had not only handed him the bottle but actively encouraged him to play with it in the manner we observed. After about two minutes of this the baby did get the nipple into his mouth at a somewhat crooked angle so that it would have been impossible to suck in his position. The mother then put the nipple into his mouth more straightforwardly and held it for him so that he might suck if he wanted to. He was still in the state of playful excitement previously described and his excited arm motions made it difficult for the mother to right the bottle in the baby's mouth. It seemed that once the nipple was in his mouth he didn't really suck, and by 2.14 p.m. the mother removed the nipple from his mouth and, with an indulgent smile in the baby's direction, said that she felt he was now very sleepy'.

The next example not only illustrates the active way in which Jerry responded to such a manipulation as being dressed, but also the fact that, even when involved in a social interaction, toys had the power to distract him. It also shows his mother's awareness of this and the ingenious and adaptive fashion in which she exploited her son's responsiveness to objects for the purpose of reducing the amount of frustration involved in a necessary procedure.

'It seemed to me that the mother dressed the baby in an extremely tactful fashion with a purposive aim of causing minimal disturbance to the baby. Just before she started to dress him, the baby was in a prone position at the side of the crib next to the wall. The mother provocatively dangled his T-shirt[1] up over the other side of the crib and said to him softly and teasingly "Come and get it." She continued to dangle it until finally the baby made his way toward it, whereupon he grasped the lower end of it and she pulled the T-shirt over his head quickly. This was done with the baby in the prone position. Once the shirt was over his head he started to fret a little and then to pivot. The mother gently but firmly placed him in the supine position. He fretted, she gave him a toy. While he kicked she pulled his overalls over his legs. Then, as he continued active, she brought him to a standing position, and, since she had so much difficulty in holding him while she drew up and fastened his overalls, she asked me to "balance" him while she finished up the dressing. Whenever he dropped his toy she picked it up for him. She worked with him gently and a good deal of the time talked to him very softly and playfully'.

From what we saw on other occasions and from everything the mother could tell us, the immediate, active, exploratory and manipulative relationship to objects was highly characteristic of Jerry at all

---

[1] A T-shirt is a cotton jersey garment, light-weight and usually gaily coloured (Jerry's was bright red). We were especially impressed with the mother's skill in arousing his interest in the shirt before pulling it over his head. As he disliked the latter procedure, it was clearly her aim to have him approach the shirt so she would not have to approach him with it. Even babies resent discomfort less if they need not feel themselves as entirely passive recipients, but have had a choice in the matter.

times. It remains for us to describe more fully the kinds of objects which were available to him throughout his day. (This also provides us with an opportunity to summarize the routine aspects of his daily life.)

As Jerry awoke in his crib each morning (usually shortly after seven o'clock and just before his father left for work) he tended to be more quiet than during any other waking time. Apparently he sometimes found the bottle over which he had fallen asleep the night before. More usually he just stretched and moved about, probably fingered the sheets and blankets, and the mother felt that he derived enjoyment from watching his parents move about in the vicinity.

Shortly afterwards he was put on the high-chair in the kitchen and given his breakfast, consisting of cereal and fruit. Thus, in addition to whatever toys one might guess his mother provided to tide him over the waiting periods, he was relating himself to a variety of tool-objects. Clothes to be put on his body, the chair to be sat on, the spoon to be fed with, the dish containing the food, etc. Thereafter he and his morning bottle (another tool-object) were put into his crib. He usually took a small amount of milk and fell asleep again. More often than not Freddy, who was up and about by then, wakened Jerry around nine o'clock. Then followed a play period which he usually spent in either the jumper-swing, or the high-chair, or both. The variety of objects he used, both those intended as toys and those that were not, was very large. He had quite a collection of rattles, rubber toys and the like, which were his own. His favourite at the time was the one his mother had made for him by tying together several old piano keys. His teddy-bear did not yet interest him though he would pat it occasionally. His brother's miniature cars, airplanes, etc., seemed to have an unholy fascination, or so it would seem from the fact that Freddy so often had occasion to defend his property rights.

It seemed that Jerry played with anything of a size convenient to his grasp, and that his play was of much the same variety with most of the toys. He enjoyed making a noise by banging things; if they were smooth or soft (like rubber or ivory or plastic) he often brought them to his mouth. While his play with one object did not differ much from that with another, he did get bored with his toys. We observed, and the mother told us, that when he had played with several for some time he became restless, threw or dropped them more often than before, and might vocalize impatiently. Unless he was also sleepy or hungry at the time, a few different toys satisfied him and he played contentedly some more.

Needless to say, neither Jerry's nor anybody else's day divides itself into portions wholly devoted to things or to people. All morning long, in fact all day long, people responded to him and he responded to them. Mother and brother talked to him, touched him, gave him toys, took toys away, created noise and movement, colour and light for him to watch, and altered his points of observation by now lifting him and now putting him down again. However, as compared to many children of his age, an especially large proportion of Jerry's social contacts employed the medium of objects. His mother dressed, diapered, fed or moved him. If not, she was more apt to hand him toys or pick up and return those he had dropped than she was to hold him or merely talk to him. Freddy swung him in the jumper-swing (high enough to make him cry if mother did not watch) or negotiated with him over toys. Apparently the only person who sometimes merely sat by him and talked to him was the father of an evening. (Even this is not certain as the mother might have described this contact thus even if toys were a part of the situation.)

At any rate, at noon-time there followed another feeding, usually consisting of mixed vegetables, soup or meat, and some fruit. Freddy ate at the same time and both children received a cooky if they had eaten all their lunch. (One gathers that this was seldom problematic in Jerry's case, as he thoroughly welcomed most food and, if anything, tended to gulp it too quickly.) After lunch he remained on the high-chair playing until he showed signs of sleepiness. From some incidental comments made by the mother, we judge that he was as likely to be playing with kitchen utensils as with proper toys. In addition to the continuation of object relations already mentioned, the noon meal provided one different kind of interaction with a thing. Eating a cooky placed in one's hand, and thus causing it to disappear, is surely different from opening the mouth to receive food, or from biting inedible toys.

When his irritability, loss of interest in toys, and bodily restlessness convinced the mother of his sleepiness, Jerry was put to bed with another bottle (he did not receive milk with lunch). This usually occurred about two o'clock. Most often he slept about two hours and awakened to another play period. Again he might spend it on the jumper (the mother thought he preferred it and said it was 'his pride and joy'), the high-chair or both. Again the mother, now engaged in supper preparations, found it not difficult to keep him interested in a variety of toys, provided he was spoken to and generally included in things that went on. The evening meal, between 5.30 and 6, was a social affair. Jerry's high-chair was pulled up to the table to draw him into the family circle. His usual meal seems quite a heavy one for so young a baby. On the day we saw him he had half a can of vegetable, half a banana, and half a can of custard pudding, which the mother considered an average for him.

152

Subsequently he was again expected to play, and usually did so for an hour or thereabouts. Except for the father's presence this play period did not differ from any of the others, though at times he played in the crib instead of being in one of his special seats. Shortly before bedtime (8 to 8.30), he experienced yet another social situation centred on a different kind of relation to the object world—his bath. While he himself was being put into the water and washed (i.e. treated as an object in a way), he was encouraged to splash and cause the water to move and make noises; also some of his toys routinely went into the pan of water with him. Then, with the comforting bottle as the last object of the day, he was put to bed for the night.

In summary, one might say that Jerry lived in a rich and varied world of things. His spontaneous interest in reaching, grasping, banging, manipulating and exploring things was recognized and encouraged by the important people in his world. His interaction with things was characterized by the intensity of his reactions. He easily became excited in his play with objects, and he tended to experience tension and perhaps anger and a sense of loss quite strongly when things dropped from his hands or were taken away (mother mentioned that almost the only times he cried when not hungry or in other physical discomfort was when Freddy took a toy from him). Thus a relatively large proportion of his physical energy and of his affect expenditure went into his interaction with things. In the light of his strong responsiveness to objects, it is important to note that he experienced less conflict or even friction with other persons in the context of using objects than do a great many babies. His mother took for granted that he would want to touch everything in sight and within wide limits allowed him to do so. Not once did we hear her say 'no' when the child handled an object, and she was very skilful in offering substitutes when it was necessary to remove something. Even Freddy seemed to have been trained to give the baby something to replace whatever he took from him though it is unlikely that he always abided by the rule.

Another thing that characterized Jerry's experience with things was the active attitude he maintained towards them. Many babies, likewise intensely interested in toys and such, spend a fair proportion of their time in looking at, touching and fingering, listening to, and perhaps licking objects or feeling them with their mouth. Jerry rarely showed a passive-receptive, absorbing, discriminating attentiveness to things. If he touched it was for the purpose of moving the object, if he brought it to the mouth it was to bite or champ it, if an interesting object was in sight but not in reach he was apt to become angry and irritated, or else to turn to something else more suited to his interests.

Jerry and His World of Persons

Jerry lived through his days in immediate and almost continuous contact with his mother. Less close but equally much a part of his day-by-day existence were his brother and his father, in that order. Other much more peripheral figures whom he yet recognized, in the sense of responding differently to them than he did to total strangers, were the paternal grandmother and some other relatives. In addition, by the time we knew him he was old enough to be frequently exposed to strangers. Our contact with him, of course, fell into this category until after we had become acquainted. Our curiosity was directed not so much at whom he knew and what these persons were like in their own right, but at the quality of the experience he had with them, the kinds of interaction that occurred. Direct observation was almost entirely restricted to his relationship with his mother, though his response to us illustrated his behaviour toward strangers, and the process of making friends. As to the rest, a far less accurate but probably grossly correct picture could be reconstructed from what the mother told us.[1]

Since the mother was by far the most important person in his life, we are content to believe that what could be learned about the relationship between these two was of predominant importance for all his interpersonal experiences at that phase of his life. It is hoped that the impression has already been conveyed that his mother was attentive and solicitous, without being overly protective or especially demonstrative. It remains to show more precisely what her attitudes were and the kinds of actions they led to as far as Jerry was concerned. We shall again begin with a portion of the impressionistic summaries written by the observers independently from one another (i.e. without exchanging their views until after the material was written up).

'Throughout the afternoon her manner with the baby and the way in which she spoke of him reflected very considerable pride in him. Although she verbalized her original disappointment in this baby's sex, it seemed to me that his vigorous, definitely male characteristics were one of the sources of pride. She spoke of the older child, Freddy, with equal warmth and pleasure, and I thought it interesting that she could be so obviously pleased with Jerry and at the same time soberly seek evidence for the fact that he is developing less rapidly than Freddy did.

'In handling the baby this mother was unhurried and gentle

[1]The brief occasions when Jerry was observed in interaction with his brother and his father closely conformed to what the mother had led us to expect, though this may have been partly chance.

154

without being overly cautious or gingerly. Her movements most of the time were fairly slow, although this effect may have partly been produced by the fact that she was always ready to interrupt procedures in order to permit the baby to carry out an action or in order to talk to him playfully in between. She tended, when dressing or undressing him or during similar occasions, to maintain a stream of soft, affectionate, playful talk. This seemed to me to be reassuring rather than stimulating most of the time. Her ordinarily low voice dropped a good deal when she spoke to the baby. Except for the fact that she tended to offer him toys or other objects to play with whenever he became restless, I thought that she was not at all stimulating with him.

'On the other hand, I believe that in her characteristically gentle way she does in many ways encourage him to independence even at this age. When he lost his balance and fell, as occurred quite frequently, she rarely did anything about it and made no sort of fuss. When on one or two occasions he encountered obvious difficulty in rolling from the supine into the prone, she watched this, verbalized her recognition of what he was trying to do, but waited for him to accomplish it by himself. Similarly she gave him the bottle to hold and let him labour with it for a long period of time rather than sticking it into his mouth (this at a time when he was no longer very hungry). She also mentioned the development of "independence" in connexion with her tendency not to rock him or hold him too much.

'Her face lit up whenever Jerry was mentioned in an especially positive way. She seems delighted by his every attribute, including what she called his "snoopiness", etc. Her tempo of movement appears medium. It was observed, however, that when the occasion demanded she could move very rapidly. An example of this was when she was preparing more formula for Jerry which was to be given to him in an attempt to get him to go to sleep. When working with Jerry she sometimes slowed down her tempo. At times she approached him slowly and gently in what could best be described as an unusually tactful way. She seemed always to have his comfort in mind. A good example of this is her behaviour in dressing him at the end of the afternoon. She is apparently aware of the fact that movement restraint is experienced by him as frustration, and she succeeds in imposing on him a minimal amount of restraint at the same time as she gives him adequate support so that he does not fall while standing or sitting. I got the impression that she is tactful with him, not simply because she does not want to get him upset, but rather that this is one of the ways in which her love for him and her respect for him are expressed.

L   155

'In her behaviour with the baby I could detect no signs of ambi-valence. She seems interested in thinking about what sort of an individual he is and has considerable respect for his rights as an individual.'

Lest this sound like too idealized a picture, let us hasten to add that in the course of our contacts with the mother we learned a little of the anxieties and limitations which, of course, she possessed. We did receive the impression, however, that these "weaknesses" affected her relationship with the baby to a minimal degree, though it is con-ceivable that this very mother may experience more difficulty later on, when her active sons reach an age of greater independence. The mother was a shy person, adaptive to demands placed upon her, and apparently seldom defiant or self-assertive. Her life was filled with re-sponsibilities some of which had come upon her rather early (a war marriage at nineteen, independent work under war conditions while her husband was overseas, two children at age twenty-four, loss of parents, and thus ties to own family, in recent past). Though she did not speak complainingly, one sensed that she missed many satisfac-tions, such as music, and activities related to other interests not shared by her husband. Her husband and in-laws seemed quite alien to her own previous style of life, and she conveyed the sense of some distance between herself and them, and perhaps a corresponding sense of loneliness. In speaking of her marriage, we heard of seem-ingly harmonious shared planning, and of mutual assistance in accomplishing work tasks. We heard nothing about simple pleasures of the kind which played a large role in the life of many mothers of our group. The fact that the mother did not once mention dances, parties or movies, does not mean that such did not occur (possibly they did), but we conclude that pleasure and diversion were either rare or somehow not as enjoyable and important to this mother as one might wish on her behalf.

Also, we thought her a somewhat fearful person, especially with respect to physical health. She spoke of cancer, of which her mother died, with great uneasiness. Freddy had been drinking more water than usual and she worried for fear he might have a sore throat which in turn might be caused by cancer (a child of her acquaintance had died from such cause within the year). These fears, though probably always present as an undercurrent, rose to the surface only on special provocation. While the adjectives 'somewhat fearful' and 'nervous' had occurred in our impressions after the long observation period, we did not then know anything about the content.

The mother experienced a severe fall on icy pavement a few days after her visit with us. She sustained shock and some painful though not serious injuries of the back and one leg. Bed rest was necessary at first, and from telephone conversations it was apparent that she had been badly frightened and worried as to who should look after the children if she were unable to do so. When our observer visited the home she still did not look well, experienced pain, and had not shaken off the fright. She told of these fears in immediate connexion with telling of the accident. Another example of both the presence of fear and its control was the following: When Freddy was an infant, she told us, she watched him very carefully when he slept to make sure 'he was still breathing'. With experience, she soon overcame this anxious watching, and in Jerry's case it never occurred to her at all.

All in all, then, we saw this mother as a shy and even pliant young woman who none the less knew quite well what her goals were and how to work towards their achievement. Though she had some broader interests, her life centred on caring for her immediate family. She thoroughly enjoyed both her children and, in addition to giving them good care, lovingly followed their progress and recorded it in a diary. Her married life, though begun after a short courtship, seemed stable and harmonious, yet hardly gay. She seemed intelligent and alert, and possessed of more tact and empathy than is common. While generally reserved, she would 'thaw out' in response to sympathetic and respectful interest, and a lively pleasure in, and admiration for, her children proved the best gateway to her confidence and acceptance.

The infinite variety of ways in which a baby and a mother can respond to one another can roughly be divided into a few categories. (*a*) Situations where the baby is in a state of need (discomfort); the mother perceives this and does something about it. (*b*) Situations where the baby is not in a state of acute need (anything from sleeping to playing contentedly), but the mother initiates an action for some reason (routine procedure such as dressing or bathing him or just the wish to pick him up to play with him). (*c*) Situations initiated by the baby, where he responds to her as a stimulus for pleasurable activity of some sort.[1] To us it appears that there is an important difference between those mother-baby relationships where a high proportion of the contacts arise from needs or wishes within the mother which are more or less imposed upon the baby (however benevolently), and those mother-baby relationships where this is rare, the majority of contacts arising from the mother's perception of the

---

[1]A real analysis would of course require subdivision of many sorts. The baby may turn to the mother for help with a goal of his own (as in obtaining a toy or being helped to a standing position); the mother may try to motivate the child so that with her guidance he experiences the activity (playing with a toy, etc.) as corresponding to his own impulse.

baby's discomfort, or in response to a definite 'invitation' from the baby.

One of the striking things about Jerry's mother was that she was so alert to his behaviourally expressed needs and wishes. Even while she gave her attention to conversation with one of us, or to housework, she seemed to notice his actions and step in to help him out or to fore-stall trouble. The following incidents, drawn from our records, illustrate the point.

'The baby was taking his bottle in the crib while the mother sat in a chair a few feet distant conversing with us. I noticed that throughout the mother kept a very sharp look-out for the baby. At one time he slightly increased activity and immediately afterward lost the nipple. He made only one sound but the mother was up like a flash and restored the bottle at once. At $2.7\frac{1}{2}$ p.m. this same sequence of events repeated itself.

'The baby was playing on the floor, close to the mother's feet, his interest at the moment centred on a small suitcase in which the mother had carried his belongings. The mother was replying to numerous specific questions about the baby's history. Simultaneously the following was observed. He became somewhat restless and uttered some squeals. The mother thereupon picked him up and held him to a standing position half leaning against her knees. He seemed more content in this position and supported himself well. His interest in the plastic handle was undiminished and he bent down, reaching for the suitcase, grabbing the handle with one hand and sort of tottering over it like a drunken traveller. The mother placed him in the sitting position again as before, and several times in a row, apparently because he was getting sleepy, he fell over toward the right side. On most occasions the mother caught him before he quite hit the floor, and each time he fell he fussed mildly but did not cry, although to me some of those falls seemed moderately severe ones.'

The baby did not need to endanger himself or become outright unhappy in order for the mother to display this kind of alertness. All observers commented on the almost automatic manner in which the mother picked up toys as he dropped them, and adjusted his position when his balance began to waver. During the afternoon there occurred a period of forty minutes during which the baby played and the mother spoke with us. The record contains twenty different instances of the mother's picking up a toy for the baby during this time. This is an underestimate, for, when at a given time the record said 'She continued picking up toys without interrupting her conversation', we counted this as one instance. At home the same thing was seen to occur.

A necessary supplement to the watchful aspect of her dealings with him is the lack of concern over minor unavoidable distress, and the way she encouraged him to overcome difficulties by himself if she judged him capable of so doing.

'For instance, while the baby was playing in the crib: from the sitting position he once more lost his balance and fell rather forcefully sideways and back, almost hitting his head at the side of the crib. One observer cried out in considerable alarm whereas the mother did not seem the least bit bothered and the baby merely grimaced briefly.

'And while the baby was crying from hunger and the bottle had been put on to heat, the mother returned to the baby and put his shirt on him while he cried very loudly. It was my impression that he resisted the procedure, especially when she tried to put the sleeves over his arms. The mother continued the procedure in her slow and calm way; she wasn't exactly forcing the baby, nor did she permit his distress to hinder her activities with him. Smilingly and quite undisturbedly she said to him, "You working up an appetite, uh?" Then she left the baby, who was still crying, and went over to the sink in order to get the bottle out of the bottle warmer.'

A lack of over-concern with respect to behaviours to which many mothers are especially sensitive characterized this mother. The areas which the mothers whom we knew in this study were most likely to invest with special importance were: cleanliness and toilet-training, bodily 'habits' such as thumb-sucking, and anything they considered to be related to sexuality. On all of these scores this particular mother was relaxed. For instance:

'As he lay there naked and the clean diaper was put beneath his buttocks, the baby's left hand reached for his penis and he manipulated it in what appeared to be a deliberate as well as rather skilful manner, making sort of squeezing and pulling motions. There was no erection and the baby's facial expression was peaceful rather than excited. The mother must have seen this activity since she was bending over him closely but she did nothing about it and made no comment.'

It has been mentioned that this mother disregarded some of the precautions concerning cleanliness which are maintained by many others. She sterilized neither water nor his eating utensils, and had no hesitation in letting him bring objects to his mouth no matter how often they had fallen to the floor. In talking about toilet-training she said that soon she would begin with Jerry, as he was able to sit up so well. She planned to proceed as she had with Freddy, and from her detailed description it was apparent that when the child objected to sitting on the pot she interrupted training for some weeks because she did not wish to 'force him'. When he relapsed in his, by then regulated, toilet habits during the week when the mother was in the hospital to have the new baby, she took this as a matter of no consequence and re-established elimination training very gradually. She also happened to express to us her attitude toward sex play among children of Freddy's age. A neighbour had become upset because the children had engaged in some such play, and angrily accused Freddy of being the one to start it. Instead of refuting the charge the mother calmly said that through other mothers she knew this to be normal behaviour, and that it would disappear again and do no harm provided no fuss was made concerning it.

In terms of the three broad categories of social interaction mentioned on p. 157, one can say that by far the largest proportion of contacts between Jerry and his mother occurred when the baby provided behaviour clues which served as signals to the mother, alerting her to a need on his part. Necessarily, numerous contacts occurred every day where the mother interfered with the baby's activities, or at least approached him in the absence of any indications of need or wish on his part. As far as we could determine, such contacts were based on the mother's understanding of what was necessary for the baby's welfare (bathing him, dressing him, taking him to the doctor, etc.) or what was necessary for the well-being of other family members (taking Freddy's toys from him, getting him out of the way when guests were present, etc.).

We have not yet spoken of the playful interactions between them which served no purpose other than immediate pleasure. These occurred often but not nearly as often as we have seen them occur with a fair number of other affectionate mother-baby couples. Characteristically, these playful interactions were most often secondary to some other more practical procedure. While dressing or diapering the baby, and on similar occasions, the mother almost always maintained a stream of low-voiced pleasant and animated conversation to which he responded with alertness. The few occasions when playful interaction took place as a primary activity (i.e. the mother was not simultaneously doing something else as well), it seemed interesting to us that she still tended to use some object as a medium for communication. The physical examination of the baby had just been completed, everyone withdrew from the crib around which three observers and the mother had been crowded. Each adult found a seat at some distance from the baby and there was a pause before the interview with the mother was resumed.

'In a very gentle manner the mother began to play with the baby. She made her fingers travel up the screen of the crib from the outside while the baby was scratching the screen from the inside. He watched the movement of his mother's hands with pleased interest. Again his breathing became the excited sort of huffing and puffing described previously, and again I received the impression that this was at least partially voluntary action, almost a kind of communication signifying pleased excitement. It occurred to me as I listened that the sound he produces resembles not only huffing but also wheezy breathing, but I continued to feel that this is the way in which he manifests excitement rather than any disturbance in the respiratory functioning. The baby briefly cradle-rocked. The mother seemed delighted at this accomplishment and said in a low tone of voice but with much pleasure "there you are".'

This example raises the whole problem of *communication* between mother and baby. At an age when speech has not yet been developed, there are none the less manifold ways in which feeling, or wish, or intention are communicated both to and by the baby. It is often quite impossible to know whether the infant intends to convey something to the mother, or whether he is even aware of so doing. Yet, certainly at the age of seven months and for some time before, many instances occur where it is quite clear that the baby wants something or protests against it, and is turning toward the mother with the intent of expressing his desire. The younger the infant the higher the proportion of interactions in which the mother 'reads' the baby's behaviour, i.e. interprets his actions to 'mean' that he is hungry, or sleepy, or bored, etc.

It would lead too far here to go into the nature of the process, well under way in Jerry's case at the time at which we knew him, by which babies begin to 'read' the meaning of their mother's behaviour, and mutual communication becomes intentional on both sides. In order to comprehend Jerry's social world it is necessary to recognize, however, that mothers differ in their ability to 'read 'the behaviour of their babies correctly, and babies differ in the clarity with which their preferences and dislikes are given behavioural expression. All observers commented that it was always easy to know what Jerry wanted and how he felt, which surely lightened the mother's task of meeting his needs. Since she happened to be an observant sort of person, conditions for good communication between the two of them were optimal. This means that it happened less often to Jerry than to many other babies that he was fed when what he needed was a chance to sleep, or that he was played with when he was restless from a stomach-ache. Correspondingly, the mother seldom felt puzzled as to what might be the matter with him. During the home visit such an occasion occurred when Jerry became restless in the early afternoon. The mother said that she would put him on the jumper-swing first. If he settled down there it meant that he had merely been bored; if he continued to fuss it meant that he was ready for his afternoon nap. On another occasion, asked if she could tell what made the baby cry, the mother said she found it easy to do so.

'When he's hungry he gives a steady cry. When he's sleepy he rubs his eyes and yawns and cries a bit. Then he rubs his eyes and yawns and cries some more. In other words it is an intermittent cry. When he is in pain he cries harder than when he is hungry.'

Therefore, she feels it is easy to tell what he needs.

Although a great deal could be added by way of description of the ways in which this mother and baby related to one another, only two additional observations will be stated, in summary fashion. The first concerns the mother's way of interpreting the baby's behaviour. It seemed to us that this mother relatively seldom consciously asked herself the question 'What does this behaviour mean?' She did not ask us on such points, as many other mothers did, but usually seemed to feel that it was self-evident. But in addition, and from spontaneous interest without specific purpose she tended to participate imaginatively in the baby's experience. When he was being quite active on her lap, reaching in every direction toward things, she said 'he wants everything', in a proud, understanding and affectionate way (as if she felt that we, the observers, should be given an explanation for his behaviour). During the physical examination the baby brought the tape-measure to his mouth and an observer commented

'that the baby liked the tape-measure which one observer had offered him to play with. The mother said with real interest in her voice "It's cold to his mouth". I thought this rather characteristic of the kind of empathy which this mother displayed frequently. It was as though she were really trying to imagine what the baby's experiences and sensations were'.

The second observation refers to the fact that, as compared with other babies of like age, Jerry's spontaneous interest was directed less intensively and less often at people, and proportionately more so at things. He responded to his mother in a thousand ways, but even while she was doing something with him, he was more apt to focus his attention on a part of his own body, on an article of clothing, or on a toy than he was just to regard his mother. This was true even more with persons other than the mother—she was the only person to whom we sometimes saw him give his undivided attention. However great the contrast between these two (she, gentle, slow, sensitive and adaptive; he, robust, out-going, vigorous, rapid and manipulative) they had in common a tendency to have their social interaction secondary to some other activity, and to have it mediated through things.

Given what has been said about Jerry and the other members of the family, we shall leave the reader to imagine the nature of his interaction with Freddy and the father. It will be remembered that the latter had brief contacts with him, did not tend to play very actively with him, but playfully tickled him, showed him toys, or just talked to him. The father did not participate in the routine care of the baby, and thus had little occasion either to interfere with him or to be the one to meet his needs of the moment. Whether he shared the mother's ability to attune his behaviour tactfully to the baby's preferences, we do not know. It may safely be assumed that Freddy could not have been able to meet the baby more than half-way even if he had wanted to. No doubt, more friction and failure of communication occurred between the two children than in Jerry's other social contacts. On the other hand, the mother told us that Jerry was especially fascinated with Freddy's behaviour, tried to be close to him, and greatly enjoyed it when his brother chose to play with him (at least at first before Freddy became too rough). The contacts with Freddy must have been an important element of colour, noise and movement in Jerry's life—and all these things he rather liked.

A young child's customary response to strange persons can be a good index of his state of well-being and security. Jerry was clearly aware of the difference between familiar and unfamiliar persons, but, according to the mother, had never shown fear of the latter. During the first few minutes in our office, all the unfamiliar observers were in sight. While they looked at him and smiled when Jerry's gaze crossed theirs, they did not come close until after some time had passed. The following episode is characteristic of what occurred in relation to each of the observers.

'While standing by the mother's knees in this fashion the baby regarded one of the observers with a very fascinated expression on his face. Most of the time he holds his mouth open. The observer smiled at him and he continued to look at her; I did not see him smile back, though his facial expression was one of pleased interest. At 1.18 p.m. the mother lifted him on to her lap again where he sat quietly and looked about very alertly, his glance frequently returning to the observer'.

The observer who was the object of this scrutiny described the same scene as follows:

'Then almost at once he looked toward me and gazed at me briefly with open mouth. He looked at me with interest but it was my impression that he had not yet made up his mind what he thought of me. The mother lifted the baby and took him on to her lap again. He looked away from us and began to bounce happily on the mother's lap, meanwhile taking looks at the central photographic light and towards the window. Again his regard returned to the observer and myself, and it seemed to me that this time his facial expression was somewhat friendlier.'

After approximately ten minutes Jerry smiled responsively at each of us and permitted physical contact without hesitation. The mother said that the main characteristic of his behaviour toward strangers was that he became temporarily less active and that he 'paid more attention', watching the stranger with a friendly, pleased interest. She thought also that he was more observant of the father and the grandmother than herself because he was so accustomed to her, i.e., she took his greater manifest interest in other people as a sign of the fact that he knew her as a distinct separate person (and she was probably correct in her interpretation). Concerning his responsiveness to unfamiliar persons, it might be mentioned that, after some acquaintance had been established, he was less differentiated in his responsiveness than are the majority of infants of this age under the same circumstances. He was equally friendly toward all three observers, did not pay more attention to one than to another, and, in fact, his behaviour with us was on many occasions much the same as that toward the mother. However, certain kinds of interaction occurred only with the mother. Moreover, when he cried or something other than play was done with him it was the mother who performed these actions. Had we attempted to dress him (or some such thing) he would most likely have responded to the novelty of the situation.

All in all, Jerry's world of people was evidently a friendly one. His contacts with people appear to have been preponderantly gratifying or comforting; the appearance of a person in his immediate environment seldom signalled pain, alarm or other discomfort. He knew what it felt like to be hurt by a person (the doctor with the needle, Freddy at his less gentle moments, and undoubtedly many other occasions of which we did not learn). Yet positive experiences—and perhaps the fact that he was so seldom away from the mother—must have outweighed these hurts, for new people seemed to arouse an expectation of something interesting and pleasant about to happen (not something to stay away from).

JERRY'S CONTRIBUTIONS TO HIS WORLD

Up to this point we have described Jerry's experience primarily in terms of what his environment was like. The quality of his responsiveness was emphasized chiefly as it influenced the manner in which his contacts with the outer world occurred. For the most part this has been a matter of factual description and inferences have been avoided. Yet intensive observation of a child in numerous situations —especially against the background of having made similar observations of many other children—brings out consistencies which are perceived as traits or characteristics of the child-personality. It is these consistencies which lend unity and individuality to the behaviour of the baby.

We shall now describe those of Jerry's characteristics which we inferred from the observed behaviour consistencies. It would be impractical to document each point by quotation from the behaviour records, not only because it would greatly lengthen this report, but but also because it would make boring reading. Moreover, some statements are the result of comparison between Jerry's behaviour and that of the other children in our group. We ask the reader to accept as a fact that each inference is based on numerous behaviour episodes reported by several observers. At the same time we ask the reader to keep in mind that these are *inferences* and not facts; the same observation might lead other students of the material to different inferences.

(a) Developmental Status

The most systematic assessment we made of Jerry's developmental level was by means of psychological tests. The Cattell Infant Intelligence Scale and the Gesell Developmental Schedules were administered. We quote from the psychological test report:

Cattell Infant Intelligence Scale:

Chronological age 7·3 months; Mental age 8·2 months; I.Q. 112 (bright average intelligence range).

Jerry passed all items at the 7 months' level, two at the 8 months' level, one at the 9 months' level and, surprisingly, three at the 10 months' level, none above. The scatter is thus moderately wide but extends above his chronological age level entirely. The distribution of successes and failures does not fall into an altogether clear pattern. His earliest failures occur in the area of vocalizations, which is in good accord with observations made throughout the afternoon. His most mature performance concerns the combined use of

165

several objects. These test findings leave no doubt that Jerry's development has proceeded in accordance with average expectations on the whole.

Gesell Developmental Schedules:

Chronological age	= 32 weeks
Mental age: Motor	= 32 weeks plus
Adaptive	= 36 weeks
Language	= 28 weeks
Personal-social	= 32 weeks

The findings on this test confirm those obtained on the Cattell test in that they describe Jerry as a youngster whose development has conformed to average standards by and large. While scatter within each area is narrow, scatter among areas is fairly wide. In the motor area he passed all items at his own age level and two out of five at the 36 weeks' level, none above. In the adaptive area he showed a similar unevenness to that shown on the Cattell test. That is, he passed all items at his own age level but only two out of five at the 36 weeks' level, whereas three out of eight are passed at the 40 weeks' level, none above. The mild retardation in the language area is clearly reflected on this test where he passed all items at the 28 weeks' level and none above. The distribution of scores in the personal-social area looks more peculiar than it is, so to speak. He passed all items at the 28 weeks' level, one out of three at the 32 weeks' level, all items at the 36 weeks' level and none above. This I am inclined to regard as an artifact because the two items failed at the 32 weeks' level referred to persistency and patience in reaching a goal. Jerry was characteristically impatient and immediate in his responsiveness, and his failures do not reflect lack of alertness or purposiveness, but rather the fact that an anger or tension reaction prevented him from carrying out the task.'

All observations of his behaviour confirmed the test results in that his skills, interests and comprehensions were either like what is normally seen in children at this age, or somewhat more mature than standards of his age. The observations also confirmed the fact that the sounds which Jerry produced (vocalizations) were less mature than the remainder of his behaviour.[1] We do not here refer to the expressive aspect of his vocalizations (an inarticulate howl can be very expressive indeed!), but to the kinds of sounds he made, and the degree of clarity and differentiation of sound he was able to achieve. It

[1]This is not considered a retardation in the sense of placing Jerry's performance below the normal range. Vocalizations and later speech are known to vary more than other measurable aspects of developmental progress, and his would have had to be very much less mature than they were to justify any question about the normalcy of his language development.

is possible to speculate that vocalizations and verbal communication do not play as large a role in the adaptation to the world, of infants for whom bodily activity and motor learning are of such predominant importance, as they do for children of a less active disposition. Or, it can be speculated that a child whose wishes are so often anticipated, who is so well understood by his environment as Jerry was without words, experiences less pressure toward learning to communicate by sounds and words than do others. Freddy's language development had been more rapid than Jerry's and the mother was well aware of this fact.

His physical development was equally satisfactory; we quote from the report of the project physician's examination:

'The baby is well developed and well nourished. His skin is thin and fine. On his back was a very faint rash resembling a mild heat rash. After he had been on his abdomen for a very short time a pressure mark was noted. Veins over the temples and adjacent areas of the head are slightly more prominent or more noticeable than usual. Anterior fontanelle did not quite admit one finger and is not at all soft. Posterior fontanelle is closed. Extremities are nicely formed. The interior of the baby's mouth was not examined since it seemed unlikely that he would readily permit such examination. *Cardiac rate*, as the baby was quite active, was 176 per minute; rhythm was regular. *Respiratory rate* was 68 per minute; rhythm was irregular; he was very active at this time. His penis and scrotum are extraordinarily small. Umbilicus is rather flat, doesn't bulge when he is brought to standing.'

(b) *Characteristics of Perception*

It will be remembered from the impressionistic summaries that all observers considered Jerry to be normally alert but not especially sensitive. A detailed analysis of his behaviour confirms this impression. In such an analysis we looked for the degree of responsiveness he showed to simple sensory stimuli (sounds, light, touch, etc.), and the degree to which the nature of his responses varied with variation in the stimulating conditions. Tentatively we have assumed that a child whose behaviour does not observably change as the conditions to which he is responding vary, is less sensitive than one whose behaviour tends to alter with even slight changes in environment.[1]

[1]It is possible to object that the differentiation of responsive behaviour may not be a direct function of the differentiation of the perceptual process itself. Tentatively we have thought that a discrepancy between these phases of the process is more likely to occur later in life, as a part of the development of the defence structure. At any rate, highly sensitive responsive behaviour presupposes sensitive perception; the reverse may or may not be true but in this discussion we have assumed that it is.

Jerry showed very little response to strong visual stimulation, e.g., when the photographic lights were turned on, though he noticed the event. He slept through exceptionally loud noises. In play he created sharp noises by banging metal objects on the metal table and seemed to be greatly pleased with noises so sharp that most babies we know would have blinked or been startled. He greatly preferred bright shiny objects to any others; it seemed that the intensity of brightness compelled his attention and that soft-coloured objects impressed themselves less upon his awareness (if he only saw them—once he held a toy it was a different matter, but he still dropped soft-coloured ones when shiny objects appeared in his field of vision). Numerous small details often noted by other babies at this age appeared not to be noted, and certainly were not responded to by Jerry. When he held a small bottle containing a pellet upside down, and the pellet dropped out, he paid no attention..He neither looked at nor touched the clapper inside the bell, etc. When he fell quite forcefully he seemed either undisturbed or grimaced briefly, when most children would have cried.

Although Jerry gave no signs of being highly sensitive with respect to any sensory modality, he did seem more so in some than in others. All observers commented that he seemed more responsive to touch than to other sensory stimulation (noted especially during physical examination, but also at other times), which fits in with the mother's report to the effect that he was a very ticklish baby. We feel on less firm ground (fewer observations) in stating that, in spite of his tolerance of loud noise, he was somewhat more sensitive in the auditory sphere than the visual one. He was seen to note the rather soft noise when the camera was turned on, and when one wished to attract his attention it was easier to do so by creating a fairly soft sound (toward which he would turn) than by other methods.

On the responsive side, we have already reported on the relative lack of differentiation. He used one toy much like another, failing to exploit the differential characteristics of each one. He behaved in much the same way toward each of three observers (which is not the case with many other babies), and in many situations behaved toward us as he did toward his mother. He had few food dislikes (no strong ones) or preferences, accepting most foods with equal pleasure.

(c) Characteristics of Tempo

In marked contrast to his mother, Jerry was on the rapid side with respect to those processes involving tempo that could be observed or learned about. He moved quickly and vigorously almost always; we never saw tentative, cautious, delicate kinds of motions on his part. He did move more slowly for a few minutes after he had been awakened but then he appeared partially drowsy. While we knew him, and according to the mother always, he ate very quickly. The fact that, in response to diet changes, he tended to develop diarrhoea (but never once was constipated) may be regarded as in keeping with a general readiness toward acceleration of function. Even his normal digestive processes were a little faster than in most babies of his age, in that he usually had four to five bowel movements during the twenty-four-hour day. His cardiac rate and respiratory rate were nearer to the upper extreme among our group of thirty-two-week-olds, though this may easily have been a by-product of his generally high activity level. His reaction time (interval between perception of a stimulus and response) was very short indeed. He typically responded at once if he was going to respond at all. Thus, in as far as his spontaneous tendencies could make it so, Jerry's experience moved at a comparatively rapid pace.

(d) Vigour and Impulse Strength

An assessment of the strength of impulse experienced by a baby is again a matter of inference. The assumption is (very tentative and provisional on our part) that children who can be seen to expend more energy in executing actions which appear primarily motivated from within (rather than by external stimulation) experience impulses with greater intensity.[1] By this criterion one would judge that Jerry characteristically experienced impulses with considerable intensity. He ate relatively large amounts and eagerly (intensity of hunger sensation?). He moved a great deal and very forcefully, not only when approaching toys, etc., but also as a self-contained, apparently pleasurable activity. When movement had to be restrained, as during dressing procedures, he fussed and protested so that the mother had to give much scope for free movement in order to forestall marked frustration-tension. (All of these may refer to impulse for bodily movement.) He brought toys to his mouth and vigorously, though briefly, champed and bit them (impulse toward oral gratification?). He was one of the few infants in our group who was seen to manipulate his penis. (This did not seem to be accompanied by tension and may not have had the quality of direct impulse gratification.) However one wishes to understand the phenomena, it is certain that Jerry's behaviour was typically energetic and vigorous.

[1]Our present speculation is that this relationship is less likely to hold at a later age when controls begin to operate.

SUMMARY

We chose Jerry for this presentation because everything we could learn concerning his development and his functioning at age seven months combined to yield a picture of harmonious, integrated, healthy development. A vigorous, actively responsive infant found himself in a rich and stimulating, yet also an adaptive and protective environment. His mother was the chief and permanent person in his life, and all vital processes (eating, sleeping, etc.) were closely connected with her physical presence in his experience. At the same time he was given a great deal of scope to engage in whatever activities he spontaneously developed. The mother not only consciously respected his preferences and dislikes with respect to foods, schedule for sleep and meals, positions, etc., but by good fortune the mother's preconceptions as to what is expected of a baby largely coincided with his natural modes of behaving. Equally fortunate was the circumstance that an infant so attracted towards things and their manipulation found himself surrounded by a multitude of suitable and available objects. Like all children, he experienced his share of pain and temporarily unsatisfied need, and found himself hindered and restrained. It was our impression that in the context of an existence basically gratifying he was less deeply disturbed by such events than are many other babies. By virtue of his sturdy organism and his supportive environment, he already had at his disposal means of overcoming tension and pain and re-establishing an equilibrium. He knew how to console himself for disappointment by turning towards a pleasurable activity instead. With respect to more basic needs, in the face of which a baby so young is necessarily helpless, his mother reliably provided appeasement.

170

Part Two

FRENCH

CASE

HISTORIES

THE FRENCH CASE HISTORIES AND SOCIAL INQUIRIES

Jenny Aubry

In December, 1951, we were asked to prepare, for the Chichester Seminar, case material concerned with child-rearing practices in France, and their influence on child development. This was a difficult task, because up to that time no studies on this topic had been undertaken in France. It was decided to use money made available by the World Federation for Mental Health, out of a grant from the United States Public Health Service, to gather, within a short period (three months), some case records of typical French families.

The research team was made up of a paediatrician with special training in child neurological development, Dr. Cyrille Koupernik; a psychiatrist with special training in the use of the Gesell test, Dr. Marcelle Geber; and a psychiatric social worker with experience in research surveys, Mme. Laurette Amado.

We had first to choose between taking a sample large enough to give statistically reliable results, and making a detailed study of a small number of families on which, perhaps, further work might be planned in the future. Having decided on the latter course, it was necessary to limit the number of variable factors very rigorously. The sample was limited to families in which mother and father were living together, with one young child, at least, in the home. The reason for this decision was the fact that the mother's first pregnancy may have an important impact on the relationship between the father and mother. For example, old, unresolved difficulties of the parents' own childhood may reappear at such a time, and may either upset the stability of the marriage or else may be worked through by the parents before the end of the child's first year.

The sample was taken from three sources, an industrial working-class community; an agricultural population in a district near to Paris; and an 'intellectual' group of parents, who were engaged in higher technical education. To limit social and economic factors in the first-named group, and because of local convenience, the sample was composed of families in which the fathers were skilled factory-workers. By excluding the unskilled factory population, many social variables were avoided, such as social instability, lack of permanent housing, poor nourishment and economic deprivation.

173

The families used in the sample were selected by the staffs of two maternity and child welfare centres, from among families with a child between one and two years of age, the child being in good physical health and of normal development, with no significant behaviour problem. An equal number of boy and girl children were included. Data was then obtained in the following respects:—

(1) Physical development of the child:

    (*a*) physical growth, neurological development, and nutrition;

    (*b*) a history of physical development and nutrition with particular reference to difficulties in assimilation and elimination, and to physical illness.

(2) Psychological development of the child: the study of development according to the Gesell scale; and an assessment of the quality of the relationships displayed by the child during the test:

    (*a*) with his mother, and her response to his behaviour, success or failure.

    (*b*) with the tester, being a stranger to the child but behaving sympathetically.

(3) Social structure of the family:

    (*a*) an account of family structure and of the interpersonal relationships between father and mother, and their attitude towards the child before and after birth;

    (*b*) in order to throw light on (*a*) above, information about the parents' own childhood experience, allowing for distortion of memories brought about by emotions. The aim was to elicit the main conflicts which the parents had gone through and their methods of solution, and in this way to throw light on the problems which might arise between parents and child.

METHOD OF WORK

The first task was to secure the co-operation of the parents to the idea of testing the child and of submitting to an inquiry themselves. Dr. Koupernik and Dr. Geber visited the family together, respectively examining the child and observing the responses of both mother and child. This procedure enabled the person giving the test to be more receptive to the child's responses and to concentrate on making a relationship with the child. Later, a discussion between the observer and the tester served to lessen the probability of subjective interpretations of test phenomena.

The inquiry by the social worker proved more difficult. A questionnaire method was discarded in favour of the more spontaneous method of personal interview. Mme. Amado was careful to stress to the parent the nature of the inquiry, and that the child had been chosen because he appeared normal and belonged to a normal family. Co-operation was given readily by all the town-mothers, and only one needed reassurance about her child's normality. Mothers in the country were far more reluctant, and many refused. The first interview was short, of from ten to fifteen minutes' duration, and took place in the clinic. Subsequent interviews took place in the home, and each urban family was visited three or four times for about one and a half hours each time. Owing to difficulties in transport, rural families were visited much less often.

On the occasion of the first home visit, the mother was seen alone. The project was explained again, and the mother asked to tell as much as possible about her child, her methods of handling him, her routine and any problems of which she was aware. At the first interview, there was practically no questioning by the social worker, but even without questioning the mothers tended to describe not only feeding, sleeping and toilet-training procedures, but also brought up the problems of their pregnancy, marital relationship, and even their own childhood. If this were not so, during the second interview, when the mother had gained some reassurance, the social worker would draw attention to the relation between the mother's handling of the child and her own childhood experiences, and this was usually enough to bring out more material. Subsequently, it was asked what the father thought of the inquiry: whether he was interested and would be willing to give his own point of view. In several cases the social worker was able to meet the father, with whom one interview was considered to be enough, since the parents would already have discussed between themselves the significance of the problems raised during the interview with the mother.

Resistances encountered with the parents, attributable to their personal difficulties, were not faced directly. Some mothers were hostile, perhaps because of previous contact with social workers who had tried to impose upon them a way of life, without understanding their personal problems. Most of the country-mothers and about half of the town ones were hostile to some extent. When the social worker sensed this hostility in the mother, she would at once acknowledge the fact that community services tended to interfere too much with family life, particularly when public money was involved, as in health insurance and so on. At the last interview some attempt would be made to broach the parents' problems, particularly by trying to show how the child's behaviour was linked with the parents' attitudes.

After the data had been collated, the team discussed the material, and tried to assess the dynamics of the family structure and the quality of the handling of the child. On the whole, the case material is not as complete as we would have wished it to be, but the team considered that a limit of four interviews should be set. This was to avoid starting a process of change in the family structure which might have undesirable repercussions if not followed through skilfully.

It is felt that this method of work gave better results than a questionnaire would have done. With the latter, it is difficult to allow for distortions caused by the parents' wish to appear better than they are; or, alternatively, if they have strong feelings of guilt, worse than they are. Moreover, questions sometimes disturb a precarious adjustment when there is a good deal of anxiety present. In one of our cases, even the careful procedure which we adopted raised anxiety in the mother, and although this was dealt with to some extent in the four interviews, the mother asked for more help and was eventually directed to a Child Guidance Clinic. .

We came to the conclusion that all such inquiries, undertaken in a brief space of time, need special care and skill to avoid distortion of data, disturbance of the adjustment of the subjects, and hostility towards the community social services. If the purpose of the inquiry is to acquire data for research, the need for care is very great indeed.

1. THE S. FAMILY

(*Urban Working-Class*)

Mme. Laurette Amado

The family consists of the mother, aged 31; the father, 36½; and their two daughters: Janine, 5 years 11 months, and Danielle, 18 months.

Since 1945 they have been living in a three-roomed flat consisting of a dining-room, bedroom, kitchen and W.C., on the first floor of a little house of which they are joint proprietors. It was a legacy from the maternal grandparents of M.S. and is fairly well furnished, for working-class people, with the grandparents' furniture. It is well kept, though nothing out of the ordinary. They have water, gas and electricity. For heating they have the cooking stove, which gives a little warmth to the dining-room, where the two girls sleep, in separate beds.

Madame S.

Born 26th November, 1920, at Bréhat, of a Breton family, is very much attached to her birthplace, where she lived with her family, including her two sisters, until the age of 18.

Her father: aged 61. Retired from the Navy as a 'master mechanic', an important position, according to his daughter. He still works as an engineer in the island boats, and enjoys very good health, but is given to drink.

He had seen service in the colonies and was often away from home. He was a very difficult character: had violent fits of rage, when he threatened and struck his wife, and terrorized his family. He was often drunk, but when sober he was kind, warm-hearted and spoilt his daughters, while remaining strict with them. He did not like them to go out, especially to dance, although this was the only distraction available on the island. He was not affectionate with them.

He is respected in the district, where he is deputy mayor, and is very religious.

Her mother: aged 58. Has been ailing for several years but never complains. At present is afraid of cancer, and as a result of this, apparently, she has suffered from 'nervous depression' since she had warts on her face in December, 1951. A very religious, good, gentle,

177

understanding woman, she has done everything for her children, and has been an 'ideal mother'. Mme. S. speaks of her with much affection and gratitude.

Mme. S.'s childhood seems to some extent to have been marred by the personality of her father, for whom she says she had no love, and the thought of him still saddens and disgusts her; but it was at the same time happy, thanks to her good and affectionate mother. Mme. S. is in close touch with her family; she writes every week to her mother who usually replies regularly every Tuesday; but the last letter was written by her father, as her mother was too much depressed to reply herself. This worries Mme. S. very much. The S. family goes on holiday every year to Bréhat for a fortnight or a month, and Janine stays there for three months.

Eldest sister: 36 years old, wife of a miner, widowed for three years. Has four children (13, 11, 7 and 3), all in good health. They live at Saint Brieuc. Mme. S. and she write to each other regularly and see each other in the holidays.

Second sister: aged 26, a widow after being married for eighteen months (her husband died of intestinal tuberculosis). She was pregnant at the time of his death and had a miscarriage. At present she is working in Paris.

The three sisters are very much attached to each other. They got on very well when they were children, without any difficulties. They used to go to dances together.

Mme. S. had a very religious education but no longer practises. She now only prays in difficult times, but does not think this right. Her childhood was uneventful except for upsets caused by her father, who, happily, was often away at sea. She has never been ill. She passed her C.E.P.[1]; was a dressmaker for three years, and then left her family because she did not get on with her father, who suggested her leaving. She took a job in Paris from 1938 to 1940, then in Rouen and Bréhat, with the same employers.

In 1941, her eldest sister, who was married by then and lived at Bizerta (her husband was in the army), asked her to go and help with her three children. Mme. S. soon had enough of it because the children were very difficult. A friend of her brother-in-law often came to the house; he made love to her, and although she did not love him, when he proposed marriage she accepted, thinking that it was a good way of getting away from her sister's, where she was acting as servant.

They went out together for four months before the marriage,

[1]Certificat d'Etudes Primaires (Primary School Certificate).

178

which took place on 23rd February 1943; there were no sexual relations before marriage. He is a 'caporal-chef', a non-commissioned officer in the regular Army.

It was a 'marriage of convenience' and 'on the rebound' for Mme. S., who had been unofficially engaged since childhood to a boy from her birthplace. They were very much in love with each other but had no sexual relations. Then while Mme. S. was away, he had a child by another woman and married, and she heard no more from him.

She is always thinking about this man whom she sees every year when they are on holiday at Bréhat; and each time it is a painful experience. She shows emotion when speaking of him, and feels guilty towards her husband because of her continuing love for the other man. Her husband knows about it but thinks it is all over. For Mme. S. this fiancé remains her ideal man, whom she would have liked to marry.

After marriage Mme. S. lived at Bizerta, in Army married quarters, until June, 1945, when she was repatriated. Her husband was often away during this period, serving with the Free French Forces, but as she was not in love with him, she did not mind this.

On returning to Paris she found her husband on leave, staying at an aunt's house. He was posted away again in December, 1945. She was pregnant then, and found herself again alone, in a flat belonging to the maternal grandparents of M.S., which the rest of the family generously let the young couple have as they possessed nothing of their own. She settled down there, alone, a long way from home, but pleased to have left Bizerta where she lived under rather difficult conditions, and also pleased to be pregnant. When her husband returned home for good they got along pretty well. She adapted herself fairly easily to her new situation.

Mme. S. speaks of herself as very timid, 'soft', nervous, sensitive and dreamy. She is certainly more of a mother than a wife. She is pleased to have two children but does not want any more as she finds they make a lot of work, and there is the future to think of.

She would very much like to go out, and go dancing, but is tied by her two little girls. She goes alone to the cinema every Saturday evening and her husband does the same on Sunday evenings, as they have no one to look after the children. She reads little, and her preference is for intimate revelations and love stories.

In short, she lives with a secret, idealized love for her unfaithful fiancé and fatalistically accepts her present situation, which is not very hard to bear.

Mme. S. is of average height, neither pretty nor plain, very vivacious, dynamic and gay. She is of average intelligence, and expresses herself well. She is well-groomed.

179

Monsieur S.

Born at Courbevoie in March, 1915.

His mother died in 1924, at the age of 30, in uraemic coma. He was then 9 years old. He has very happy memories of her, and must have been very much attached to her. He was an only son, and spent his early childhood with her alone, as his father was in the 1914–18 war, and even after that, was often away from home. She was kind, gentle and affectionate, but of strong character: a woman who put up with her husband's misconduct in silence.

His father: aged 64. A sheet-metal worker, who lives at Le Mans. Since his wife's death, he has never bothered about the son, even financially. In all this time he seems to have given him no more than seventy francs, for which the son has latterly reproached him.

Three months after his wife's death, he got married again to a war widow with three children, with whom he had been associating for a long time. Moreover, he was with her when his wife passed into coma, and the son, who was with her when this happened, has never forgiven his father for it.

The new wife was arrogant and well-off, the owner of several properties; she was not affectionate, and M.S. could never call her 'mummy'. He does not like her.

M.S. had very little contact with this part of the family. He stayed with them for two summer holidays when he was 9 and 10, and for a fortnight before leaving for Indo-China at the age of 18. They very rarely write to each other. They came at the New Year after a letter from M.S. to his father reproaching him for not taking any notice of his grandchildren, but even then they did not bring them any presents.

M.S. was brought up by his maternal grandparents after his mother's death. They were butchers at Courbevoie and owned the house where the S. family is now living. They were very kind and affectionate, and were fond of M.S., who reminded them of their daughter. They both died in 1943, of old age.

M.S. was brought up with an uncle, his mother's brother (now a butcher), and an aunt, now married to a director of Citroën's. They both apparently treat M.S. more or less as a 'failure', or at any rate he feels socially inferior to them. Mme. S. speaks of them as 'very rich people' who treat her husband as a poor relation, and try to avoid him. According to his aunt, M.S. was a demanding, difficult child.

M.S. passed his C.E.P., then worked as an apprentice butcher with some friends of his grandparents. Then, at 18, with the consent of his father, he joined the Army and was in an Infantry Regiment until 1945. He was in Indo-China from 1933 to December, 1938. This was a time of great adventures which he relates freely in his family circle. He went through the 1939 war, was taken prisoner in France and escaped; he hid in Brittany, but managed to get to North Africa where in 1943 he joined the Free French Forces. He went through the Tunisian, Italian and French campaigns, landed on the Côte d'Azur, won several decorations, including the Croix de Guerre, was mentioned in dispatches, and was wounded twice in the knee.

He intended to make a career of the army but was released in 1945 with the credit of fifteeen years' service instead of the twelve years seven months he had actually served. He has very happy memories of all this active period, as well as pride in his decorations.

On his return to civil life, he was for several months in a trade training centre at Levallois, to learn sheet-metal working. At present he is a welder in a small factory; he has had five or six changes of job since 1945 but does not like changing. He worked at the Simca Motor Works on the assembly line, but much to Mme. S.'s regret, as the job was well paid, he had to leave because the pace was too fast and too tiring. Had twenty-one days' unemployment last winter, but says that he was not worried as he managed all right—he went to work at a butcher's. He is very sure of himself, knowing that he can face up to every situation and get through all right.

M.S. is gentle and affectionate with the children and with his wife. He is a 'family man', liking to help in the house, do the shopping, help in the kitchen (though he does not cook), do odd jobs, re-decorate, and act as handy man about the house. He often plays with his daughters, of whom he is very fond. He would like to have more children, especially an 'heir'; never scolds, seems patient, quiet and understanding.

He says he had no difficulties in his childhood apart from family circumstances. Worked well at school and as an apprentice; employers have always been pleased with him. He is not difficult over food, but likes everything.

M.S. does not return home for lunch, he takes his meal with him and eats it in the canteen. When he returns, about 7.30, he plays with his children, has his meal, helps his wife, goes to bed and smokes his pipe but does not read. He day-dreams, probably, as he sleeps very little (four hours); when awake, he lies in bed and smokes.

Mme. S. says he drinks, but tries to hide it. She thinks he started drinking in the army. When she knew him at Bizerta, he was already a drinker; she tried to stop him, but it was impossible. Neither gentle nor reproachful treatment can prevent him from slipping into a café in the evening before returning home. He does not drink at home; they never have any wine at table because they cannot afford it, according to Mme. S.

He is weak-willed and as a result is easily led. For about six months when Mme. S. was pregnant for the second time, that is, in the winter of 1949–50, her husband began to drink a lot, very often returned home drunk, and became violent towards his wife. Mme. S. thinks it was caused by the fact that he did not get on with her younger sister, who was living with them at the time. She then threatened to leave her husband, which seems to have brought about a marked improvement in his behaviour, and this, coupled with the sister-in-law's departure, restored a peaceful atmosphere to the home. Since this time, he has still been frequenting the café, but in moderation.

Mme. S. puts up with her husband in spite of this great failing, but she does not love him. He has no physical attraction for her (although she says he is good-looking), she does not like kissing him, nor is she pleased when he shows affection towards her; she does not enjoy sexual relations, and is frigid. He is not her ideal man, the one who remained behind at her home. She thinks one has to pay for the stupid things one does in life and put up with the consequences.

M.S. is very fond of sport, went in for cycling and walking races before the war. Now he goes to football matches on Sundays, but his wife cannot go with him because of the children, whom she takes out while he is at them. For the summer holidays they all go to Bréhat, to Mme S.'s parents. M.S. is very fond of his in-laws, and speaks of his mother-in-law with much affection. He would like to stay down there always and work there, but Mme. S. does not want to as she thinks the life is too hard.

The intimacy of their married life seems very much limited by Mme. S., who spends most of her time with her daughters (she is practically the slave of the younger one). She works in the house (her husband thinks she does too much), and day-dreams like a young girl. M.S. works, goes to the café, does odd jobs in the house, plays with his daughters and goes to matches. He gives his pay regularly to his wife, who manages the budget.

M.S. is of average height, an 'athletic' type, dark, healthy, pleasant, amiable; he says himself that he has a cheerful, unworrying disposition. He takes things in his stride without bothering too much, nor worrying on account of his family.

He is very gentle with the children, and willingly looks after them and the home in general. He has a good opinion of his wife's character and disposition but thinks she works too hard in the house. She looks after her children well.

Janine

Born at the Kilford (Courbevoie) Maternity Home on the 1st March, 1946. Easy pregnancy, a wanted baby, whether a boy or girl, though the husband hoped for a girl.

> Born at full term, a quick, easy confinement (2 hours 30 minutes).
> Weight: 2 kg. 850 gm.; cried immediately.
> Breast-fed up to fourteen months; two feeds towards the end; no feeds during the night; Mme. S. fed the baby at any time when she cried.
> Normal development.
> Walked at sixteen months; swaddled up to five months.
> First words: a little late, now is very talkative.
> Cleanliness: enuresis up to five years (stopped after measles).
> Sleeps well, eats well, no difficulties at all.
> Still sucks her thumb, her parents tease her about it.
> Chicken-pox at nine months.
> Operation for tonsils and adenoids in 1949.
> Measles in 1951.
> Good health, a big child, strong, good colour.
> Present weight: 22kg. 700 gm. Height: 1 m. 14 cm.
> Goes for three months' holiday to Bréhat, where she loves bathing.

At the time of her little sister's birth, she was away in Bréhat for three months. Mme. S. never told her she was pregnant. Janine never asked any questions, even after the birth. They simply told her that they had bought a little sister and that seems to have satisfied her. Mme. S. said she was too small to understand these things and admits at the same time that she would not have dared to tell her.

Mme. S.'s parents never discussed questions of sex with their children; Mme. S. learnt about such things at school. She thinks she will enlighten her daughters when they ask questions.

Janine is a very sensitive, affectionate child, she cries easily (sobs for a long time), sulks, hides under the table for ten minutes when she is scolded, then starts playing again. She is not shy, is playful, careful, very tidy with her things, but has no 'fads'. Is obliging, loves to play with her sister, of whom she seems not to have been jealous, although she may perhaps be so. She also plays with a boy who lives near by.

She plays a lot with her doll, is very fond of writing, and drawing. Is a greedy eater; is very timid, and dares not go to the W.C. alone. Her mother reasons with her but it has no effect. She likes school very much and works well, getting good marks; is more afraid of her mother than of her father ('Daddy is kinder'). She is slapped when Mme. S. gets irritated ('it relieves her feelings'); her chief punishment is to be sent to bed.

Mme. S. tries to bring her up by gentle treatment, and says that she has never had any trouble with this daughter, who is very vivacious, full of fun, and talkative.

Danielle

Born at the Kilford Maternity Home on 21st August, 1950. Mme. S. did not want a child, but resigned herself as soon as she knew she was pregnant. She was disappointed it was a girl.

A difficult pregnancy. Mme. S. was not well the whole time; had constant vomiting up to four months. About the eighth month, she suffered from cystitis, and was treated with methylene blue. A strain on the mother's part caused the baby to move round; it was put back into position again at the Kilford.

Confinement complete in thirty-six hours; injections were given to quicken the dilatation of the uterus; anaesthetic for the actual delivery; no instruments used. Mme. S. says that she would be afraid of child-birth now.

> Born at term.
> Weight: 3 kg. 500 gm.; cried immediately.
> Breast-fed for three months—six feeds; no feeds in the night. Then Mme. S. had a breast abscess, too much milk, and the baby was weaned; Mme. S. was very much upset about it. Bottle-fed (formula) up to five months, then cow's milk which suited the baby very well.
> Smiled: at three months
> Walked: at seventeen months.
> First words: at eight months; repeats everything but still does not make up sentences.
> Present weight: 11 kg. 450 gm. Present height: 81 cm.
> Good, regular appetite; eats everything without any difficulty, the mother is not worried on this score; Danielle eats at table with her parents.

Sleeping: Very difficult; wakes and cries every night (eleven times). Every time she wakes up she cries for her dummy which she has had from the age of eight days; never goes off to sleep without it, nor without being rocked. The mother picks her up in the day and in the night and rocks her for five or ten minutes, half an hour or even an hour. Is in bed from eight o'clock at night to eight in the morning.

She has nightmares, screams and talks. The mother is distressed by these proceedings, which wear her out, but does not know exactly when they started. At ten months, a sedative and soluble calcium were given for two or three months, but at the end of that time they were no longer effective.

Danielle is still swaddled at night because of the cold. She gets uncovered in the night, but is not fastened down in bed. She was swaddled during the day up to five months.

Cleanliness: Wets her bed at night, and now and then her clothes. Uses her pot regularly in the morning, and has done so since she was about seven or eight months old. The mother thinks it is still not late for her not to be dry and waits patiently for her to become so.

She gets very angry, stiffens herself and screams; this gets on her mother's nerves, and makes her want to slap her; but she does not always do so except at the end of the day, when she is tired. Danielle tends to be very grumpy, and is pleasant only with her sister; she smiles very little, knits her brows, always says 'no', throws everything down, breaks everything; a very difficult child, and independent, except towards her mother, whom she will not leave—hence she has frequent fits of temper.

She never cries, and never wants to kiss anyone, which annoys her mother who likes girls to be affectionate, as her elder child is. She hopes that the little one will become so, and tries to kiss her, which produces screams. Altogether a very demanding child, whose mother seems to be a slave to her. She is greedy, especially for chocolate, which is used as a reward. She is said to take after her father in physique and character.

Mme. S. says that children must be 'trained', they must not be allowed to do as they wish. She tries to speak to them gently, to remain patient, but in fact, her nerves are soon on edge and she gives in when the children try her for too long. She does not understand why the elder child has been so easy to bring up from every point of view, and why the second is so difficult; thinks she has less patience now because there are two of them. She does not wish to have any more children—Danielle has been too much for her.

Danielle would be a pretty little girl if she were good-tempered, but during the three interviews she was very grumpy, demanding and bad-tempered.

Janine is a nice-looking girl of six, with a lot of wavy hair. Her parents only find fault with the shape of her mouth, because her upper teeth protrude a little. She is pleasant, smiling, not shy, very natural and unaffected in manner.

Mme. S. was very welcoming and confiding; a little embarrassed by having revealed her innermost secrets. She asked me not to speak to her husband about his tendency to drink, which he does not wish to admit. She seemed to be a nervous, restless, anxious woman.

M.S. was pleasant, willingly relating all his adventures, going to look for his military papers, citations and decorations, but with no excessive vanity. He showed me the photo of his mother as well. He seemed to be a well balanced man, content with his lot, or wishing to convey this impression.

To sum up, this is apparently a united household; it seems that the family spirit which the two parents have developed, should ensure its stability.

EXAMINATION OF DEVELOPMENT

Dr. Marcelle Geber

Danielle S. Born 21st August, 1950.
Examined 10th February, 1952. (17 months old).

The examination was carried out in the dining-room where Danielle's bed is, together with that of her sister, aged six. This room opens off from the kitchen and is well kept.

While we asked Mme. S. a number of questions, Danielle was on her knee and the elder child stood beside her.

Mme. S. told us that her elder daughter has developed very well, that she showed no jealousy when Danielle was born, that she spends a lot of time with her and helps her to develop.

The children play a lot together and the elder never shows any impatience. She is pleased to come down to the level of her little sister. Her mother had not told her beforehand about the baby; she was staying with her grandparents, and when she returned, her mother told her that she had bought a little sister.

Danielle was born at term, developed without any difficulty. But she was a difficult character—grumpy, demanding, bad-tempered, not affectionate. She uses her right and left hands equally well. Her mother does not check her. She seems equally attached to her father and her mother; and loves children.

Mme. S. answered all the questions very simply and pleasantly. She seemed calm and relaxed, yet gave the impression of being dissatisfied. Danielle, who was on her knee, began to get impatient and her sister brought her toys. Then she got down from her mother's knee and played with her sister.

The family environment seemed satisfactory.

Appearance

Danielle has a good physical appearance. She is chubby, rosy-cheeked, has a smooth skin, her mucous membranes are in good condition, her black hair is silky, her eyes are alert and interested.

She walks well, does not run, does not climb up or down stairs, as her mother thinks she is too small and is afraid of her falling. She plays in the room with her sister, but her mother does not let her go anywhere else without her yet. She seems very confident with her mother and her sister.

She accepted us readily, looking at us and smiling. She came towards us as soon as we began to give her the test objects.

TEST.

She was immediately and spontaneously interested in the test material. She built a tower with two cubes straight off, tried unsuccessfully to make a bigger one, then again made the one with two.

She accepted each different test, one after the other, and did them with pleasure. She did the test sitting on her mother's knee, up against the dining-room table. Her sister stood near her.

During the test, she gave all her attention to the objects, showing an intense interest in them all. Her interest was greatest when she was looking at the picture book; she said several words, stroked the pictures, turning especially towards her sister. As soon as she was given the ball she played with her sister.

The test was uniform and lasted half an hour.

(1) *Development*

Corresponds to the chronological age of the child, which is now seventeen months. D.Q.=101.

(a) *Motor*

Locomotor development: she walks well, rarely falls, does not run, does not climb the stairs. (It should be noted that there is not much space, the room is small and full of furniture. Outside, she goes in her pram or gives her hand to her mother. Her mother does not let her try to climb the stairs.)

She can seat herself on a little chair and climb on to an adult's chair. She walked inside the 'ballon' (movable frame).

Her locomotor development is that of a child of seventeen months. L.Q.=99.

Manual dexterity: Danielle is right-handed. Normal prehension. She quickly grasped the lozenge between her thumb and index finger. She turned over two or three pages at a time, and threw the ball.

N   187

Her development as regards manual dexterity corresponds to that of a child of eighteen months. M.D.Q. = 105.

(b) Adaptivity

Danielle was perfectly well able to make use of her motor development to carry out certain actions.

She built a tower with two cubes, put ten cubes in the cup, took the lozenge in and out of the bottle, scribbled spontaneously, put the square in the form-board.

Her adaptivity is that of a child of seventeen and a half months. A.Q. = 102.

(c) Language

Expression: Danielle has a vocabulary of about twenty words, said 'ball', combined two or three words spontaneously. She seemed to talk a lot to her sister.

Her language expression is clearly in advance of her actual age: twenty-one months—E.Q. = 122.

Comprehension: She picked out the pictures, talked while looking at them, but did not carry out instructions. Some backwardness was noticeable here. Her level is about sixteen months. C.Q. = 94.

(d) Personal—Social

Danielle feeds herself to some extent, is clean, asks for attention when she needs it, carries about a bear or a doll, repeats words. She does not pull toys along. Here again her sister seems to contribute to her development, which corresponds to that of a child of eighteen months, nine days. P.S.Q. = 107.

(2) *Behaviour*

(a) *Towards the objects:*

All the objects interested her and she accepted them all with pleasure, and tried to do the test straight away. Her interest was kept up without any break from the beginning to the end of the test. She cried when the last object was taken away from her and especially when, seeing the box closed, she understood that the test was over.

(b) *Towards the tester:*

She made but little use of the tester. She took with pleasure the toys that she gave her, and accepted the fact that she took them away again provided she gave her others; but she never addressed her, either by speaking to or smiling at her.

(c) *Towards her mother:*

She was on her knee, therefore had her back turned to her. She did not use her very much, but on two occasions, when she was putting the lozenge in the bottle, and when she had the book, she turned to her and spoke and smiled at her.

When, at the end of the test, she got into a temper, her mother succeeded in calming her very quickly.

(*d*) *Towards her sister:*
She uses her sister the most. She talked to her, when showing her the pictures in the book and scribbling; she held out the cubes to her and threw her the ball. She smiled at her and showed her what she was doing.

(3) *The Mother*

It was also interesting to observe the mother's and sister's attitudes throughout the test.

The mother was interested by the test. She watched the child, smiled when she succeeded and encouraged her if she failed. She gave the impression of wanting to take part, but remained calm, did not appear to be annoyed, and did not jostle the child.

The sister, standing by Danielle, was very interested, watching everything she did, and if she could not manage something, wanting to show her how. Danielle looked at her and laughed. The mother very gently told her to leave her little sister alone.

Conclusion

Danielle's development is normal and even distinctly advanced in respect of language, expression and social reactions. The elder sister seems to play an important part here.

Locomotor ability is not commensurate with the child's other development, but seemingly this is due to the small amount of space the child has to move around in, and to the attitude of the mother, who is afraid of the child hurting herself.

The family environment, ties of affection between mother and child, and between the two sisters, contribute to this satisfactory development and behaviour.

PHYSICAL EXAMINATION

Dr. Cyrille Koupernik

Danielle S. Born 21st August, 1950.
Examined 28th January, 1952 (17 months old).

Previous History

Second pregnancy. Madame S. has a daughter of 6, in good health.

Previous history shows nothing pathological, either on Mme. S.'s side (she is 31) or that of M.S. (37), a welder.

Pregnancy: A rather troublesome pregnancy, more so than the first. Mme. S. suffered from cystitis, and the baby changed position during the pregnancy; in fact moved *in utero* more than her sister.

Confinement: In the Municipal Hospital at full term of 9 months. The baby weighed 3.000 grs.

Mme. S. had great pains for 36 hours, had analgesic injections on four occasions. No anaesthetic used.

At birth, the baby's head presented, no forceps.

Danielle cried immediately. No cyanosis at birth.

During the first days: did not develop cyanosis, but after the third day she had severe jaundice, which only lasted a few days.

She had no sucking or swallowing difficulties nor abnormal muscular tone.

Development

The mother thought she smiled at a human face at about 4 months. Able to follow things round with her eyes at this age. Held her head up and sat up without support at the normal time (no exact date).

Walked, holding on to somebody's hand, at about a year old; and had been walking alone for several days.

Voluntary prehension developed early.

She has been masticating for several months.

Cut her first tooth at 8 months.

Bowel cleanliness from the age of 16 months. She sometimes asks when she wants to urinate in the daytime, but is not yet clean at night. (Sphincter training began at about 16 months.)

Said 'papa' at about 8 months.

From the age of 16 months she has understood certain words and the first names of members of her family.

From the age of 16 months could express in words her desire to urinate or go out, and the fact that she was hungry.

Several days ago she said three words together: '*Ah non, alors*' (Oh, no!).

She began to be interested in her teddy-bear at the age of 1 year, and in her doll at 16 months.

She has always been looked after by her mother.

Never had any illnesses, any otitis, diarrhoea, vomiting, head injuries, infectious diseases, nor convulsions. Vaccinated successfully against smallpox at the age of 2 months.

Present Behaviour

Danielle walks with little quick steps, putting aside her frame. She does not run; she climbs stairs if she is held by the hand.

Her prehension is good, uses a pencil to scribble, can use her right hand and left hand equally well.

Play: She has not played with her hands for a long time. Plays with bricks and with her teddy-bear, loves tearing up paper, looks with interest at picture books, and in particular looks for pictures of cats.

She still throws things about a lot, but does not destroy things.

Comprehension and Language:
She understands practically all the everyday words and simple instructions (e.g. 'come here').

She readily takes her mother's hand to show her something or to get her to give her something she wants.

She does not use baby-talk any longer but repeats words easily.

She knows about thirty words.

She calls herself by her first name, slightly altered.

It is uncertain whether she recognizes herself in a mirror.

Habits:
She sleeps in a room with her sister.

For a little time she has been afraid of the dark, waking up in the night and crying.

She is also afraid of doctors; and of burning herself.

Is not afraid of falling, loves water.

Eats everything with relish, without any special preference.

She sometimes gets into a temper but never becomes breathless.

She is rather shy with strangers.

She does not show any marked preference for one or other of her parents; she adores children.

She rocks rhythmically when she is just falling off to sleep.

Does not suck her thumb.

Physical Examination

Weight: 11.200 kg.

Circumference of head: 46 cm.

Good state of nutrition.

Mucous membrane in good condition.

No skin troubles.

Muscular tone: normal, i.e. hypotonic within normal limits.

The angle of extension of the lower leg on the thigh (in flexion on the pelvis) is 150°.

Flexion of the wrist over the forearm does not exceed a right-angle.

Swinging of the arms is normal.

The tendon reflexes are normal on both sides.

The plantar skin reflex equivocal on both sides.

Conclusion: a normal child.

2. THE L. FAMILY

(Urban Working-Class)

Mme. Laurette Amado

The family consists of the mother, 20 years old; the father, 23; their son, Alain, 15 months; and their daughter, Monique, 2 months.

They live in one room, on the ground floor of a large building in Courbevoie—a room 3 metres by 2 metres 50 (10 ft. × 8 ft.), with an extension 1 metre long by 2 wide (3 ft. 6 in. × 7 ft.), forming a kitchen.

There is no other accommodation apart from an alcove in the passage for hanging things. The W.C. is also in the passage, and is for the use of all the tenants. The room is very pleasantly arranged, and very clean. It was redecorated when they moved in. They have modern furniture: a 'cosy', a cupboard, a very small kitchen table, two chairs, a stool, Monique's bed, and, folded up in a corner, Alain's bed.

There is water, gas, electricity, and central heating. A window looks out on to a small yard. The room is rather dark: they have to have the lights on nearly all the time. The place is really the porter's lodge. Mme. L. does not have to perform the duties of caretaker, except for cleaning the stairs once a week and putting out the waste-bins every morning.

They pay two hundred francs rent a month. Heating is extra.

Madame L.

Born April, 1932, at Puteaux; but she has always lived at Courbevoie in a little flat of two rooms and a kitchen, where her parents are still living.

Her father: 41, employed in a paint shop. He is very pleasant, a good father and affectionate. He is in good health.

He was called up in 1939, and a prisoner in Germany until 1945. On his return found it difficult to re-adapt. He had changed greatly in character; at first seemed somewhat depressed, but less so now. He has tended to isolate himself since his return, goes fishing or walking, is not as cheerful as before, does not drink, does not smoke; before the war he was very lively and gay.

Her mother: 38, in good health, except in December, 1951, when she suffered from *erythaema nodosum*; she is still a little tired. She was an upholstress until the birth of her second daughter in January, 1949.

She is a practising Catholic, and is of a youthful disposition, gay, gentle, kind, understanding, and affectionate.

She is very particular about cleanliness, and thinks that she alone can do things the way they should be done (she used to re-do things that her daughter had done when she helped in the house, and criticized the way she had done them); everything has its own place, which must not be changed; slippers must be worn indoors so as not to spoil the polish.

Like her husband, she had difficulties on his return from captivity; but with both of them, these troubles were hidden, and there were never any scenes or recriminations. However, the daughter realized the position, and the mother has since talked to her about it.

Mme. L.'s parents are a very happy couple, and Mme. L. loves them both very much. As they do not live far apart, they see each other at least three times a week.

Her maternal grandfather died in 1947 (prostate), aged 81. He had been a widower for a long time; Mme. L. never knew her grandmother. He was a taxi driver, and lived in the same house as the parents of Mme. L., who was greatly attached to him. He used to spoil her a lot, took her for rides in the car.

Her sister: 3 years old; born in January, 1949.

The parents may not have been very pleased about having a child so long (seventeen years) after the other one—particularly the father, the mother says she was happy about it at once—but they quickly accepted the fact.

She is somewhat delicate, was operated on for tonsils and adenoids last year, and has otitis. She is 'dainty, sharp, intelligent', and has apparently developed normally, very quickly learning to talk. She was put on the pot from eight months onwards; was clean at eighteen months, but used to wet the bed.

Mme. L. is very fond of her little sister, and used to look after her before her marriage. She immediately accepted her advent, which her mother told her about at the beginning of her pregnancy.

Mme. L. seems to have spent a happy childhood, although disturbed by the absence of her father during the war. She was only about eight years old when her father went away, and thirteen when he returned. This period was somewhat difficult, emotionally and materially, the mother by herself having to provide for the household. Mme. L. was much indulged by her grandfather at this time. He adored his granddaughter.

Without being in easy circumstances, the family lived comfortably, the father and mother both going out to work. Now they have only the wages of one to live on, and find things a little difficult, but Mme. L. tries to help by giving them things they need.

Mme. L. is in very good health. She was never ill, except for measles and chicken-pox. She continued to wet her bed until eleven years of age; menstruation began at fourteen.

She gained her C.E.P. (Certificat d'Etudes Primaires), then did three years dressmaking, but did not get her C.A.P. because she failed in one question. She became an apprentice with Worth, where she worked until the end of her first pregnancy. She liked her trade very much, and the firm where she worked. However, she thinks that at that time she became 'envious' and wanted more clothes. The opulence of Worth's turned her head a little, but she does not regret it because she became more mature through this experience. She had many friends in the workroom and at school, and has kept in touch with quite a number of them. She likes to mix with other people, and forms easy and loyal friendships.

She is very fond of sport; was a member of a women's athletic team, has even taken part in competitions in Italy, at Nice, and in many provincial towns. Very fond of swimming. Her parents allowed her a great deal of freedom, having every confidence in her. She 'told her mother everything'; even now, she has no secrets from her.

When she was nearly eleven years old, her mother gave her sexual instruction, explaining things to her simply; she said she was never embarrassed by these subjects, which she considered quite natural. She told her about menstruation and about babies, and she will follow the same procedure with her second daughter.

Mme. L. helped her mother with the housework, but the kitchen was her special domain. She has always liked doing housework, and cleaned her own room, had certain things to do that no one else must touch, and ironed her clothes. It appears that the only trouble that arose between mother and daughter was in connexion with the cleanliness of the house, each wishing to do things according to her own ideas, and neither wishing to give way to the other. They used to quarrel 'like cat and dog' about this.

Mme. L. thinks that at that time she was rather unkind, quick-tempered and obstinate; that she said unkind things to her mother, was very overbearing, a little too much the 'only child'. Now, especially since her marriage, she has become gentler, but she still considers herself somewhat 'bossy' and over-careful, though not as much so as her mother. She does not like to see things untidy, and her cupboard is very neatly arranged; she folds up her little boy's clothes as soon as they are finished with, and does the same with blankets, sheets, etc.

Mme. L. was not thinking of marriage when she got to know her husband through one of her friends, who was having a flirtation with a young man who used to go about with another boy. They talked to each other one evening, when the four of them met, and Mme. L. continued to meet the boy on several occasions, but just as a friend. Then he enlisted in the Army, and asked Mme. L. to write to him, which she did, and they saw each other again when he came home on leave. They kept up the correspondence while M. L. was in Indo-China for a year and a half. When he returned they discussed marriage, but as something far away, considering themselves to be rather young, without jobs, and without a home. They became lovers, and Mme. L. became pregnant. Both their families were very understanding and they married four months later, on 3rd June, 1950. It was a civil ceremony, as M. L. is not a Catholic.

Mme. L. was greatly embarrassed, and blushed, at having to disclose that she was pregnant before her marriage; she feels that she was to blame for not having waited until then. She is very happy, loves her husband very much, and even though she was a little upset at becoming pregnant so soon, and twice in such a short time, she has accepted it very well. She likes to busy herself about the house, and with her children, never feeling that things are too much for her. She manages everything quite easily, sees her friends, goes out, and sews for herself, for the children and even for her little sister. Her one great desire at the moment is to find an apartment of at least four rooms, so that she can have one to herself. The couple lived for a month with her parents-in-law, when they were first married, until her father-in-law found this room for them to live in.

Mme. L. does not want any more children, now that she has a son and a daughter. She was disappointed at having a boy, and is pleased now to have a girl. She wanted to have girls chiefly so that she could dress them nicely—she is very much attracted by pretty things. She wants to provide for the children well so that they will not have to work in a factory, and thinks that she would only be able to do this for two children.

Mme. L. is of medium height, and slim. She is very pretty, fair, pleasant, intelligent, very congenial, and refined; she is dressed stylishly and looks smart and neat. She lives simply; says she has no problems. She enjoys life, needs plenty of physical exercise and of friendship; is not a dreamer. She likes to go out, to go dancing, walking, and to the cinema. In the evenings she reads, mostly detective novels and fashion magazines, and plays cards.

She considers that she was well brought up, and would like to bring up her children in the same way. She received a religious education, but does not practise any more. She will have her children baptized

195

in order to avoid difficulties later on, should they wish to marry a Catholic.

Monsieur L.

Born 2nd December, 1928, at Bagneux. He is a sheet-metal worker in a large aircraft factory.

His father: 48, chief clerk at the town hall of Courbevoie. He is very kind, affectionate, cheerful, is healthy and does not drink.

His mother: 44, a typist; very charming and gay.

They are very happy together and like going out. They are quite well off; as both have good jobs they live very comfortably, and every year they go to the Côte d'Azur for their holidays. They have a nice, well-furnished flat of four or five rooms. Mme. L. gets on very well with her parents-in-law, who accepted her without trouble.

His brother: 22, a barman, unmarried, lives with his parents. He joined the Army at 18, was wounded in Indo-China, and returned to France in 1948.

He makes fun of everything, is careless, extravagant, unstable, but pleasant and gay. He did not like school, would not study, and failed his C.E.P.

A second brother died eighteen years ago, of poliomyelitis, at the age of 5.

M. L. was at school up to his C.E.P., which he did not pass because of his bad memory, he says. His father would have liked him to take his baccalaureate, but he himself preferred to go to work straight away. He did an apprentice training course to be a sheet-metal worker.

He joined the army at 18 for a three-year term of service, but had to stay for four years, because he was in Indo-China at the end of his term, and there was no boat returning to France. He was a parachutist, first of all in North Africa, then for a year and a half in Indo-China, in the same sector as his brother and many of his friends who joined up at the same time. He enjoyed this period of adventure, which seems to have matured him. He finally came home in November, 1949, and married in June, 1950.

M. L. has always worked as a sheet-metal worker, but with several firms which he left, not voluntarily, but of necessity. He is very fond of sport; goes in for wrestling and judo, football, athletics, swimming, cycling (used to go in for races, but has stopped this since his marriage for lack of time). There are facilities for judo and football at the factory.

He had a happy, uneventful childhood with his parents, who got on well with each other, and who took a lot of trouble over their children, trying to make them happy. Their father regrets not having been able to make them do better with their studies, and wants to help his grandchildren to have professional careers. M. and Mme. L. agree with this, and have confidence in him.

M. L. is quiet, rather shy at a first meeting, but afterwards confident, gay and joking. He is very affectionate towards his wife and children. He likes to be with friends, to go dancing, to the pictures (adventure films), to read (detective novels), to play games; but he is also quite happy to stay at home listening to the wireless and occasionally helping his wife, although usually he does not help in the house or with shopping. His wife does not want him to, moreover, as he is not very good at this sort of thing, not being careful about what he buys, or the price.

It is therefore Mme. L. who manages the family budget, and her husband always gives her his pay. She does not keep accounts; but finds she has plenty to live on, and is never in difficulties though she buys everything she wants for herself, her children or her husband (she buys his suits). She is even able to buy useful presents for her mother.

M. L. does not either drink or smoke, and always comes home at the same time. He works a forty-eight-hour week (eight hours overtime), and likes his work. He has no political activities—'politics do not interest me'.

He is of medium height, slim, and dark, with a small moustache; he is less frank than his wife, because of his shyness.

Alain

Born after full-term pregnancy, 12th November, 1950, at the Kilford Maternity hospital. The mother had not wanted this pregnancy, but hoped for a girl, so that she could dress her prettily. She vomited frequently for the first eight months.

> The baby cried immediately;
> Weight, 3·100 kg.
> Breast-fed up to three months; six feeds, with a bottle of sweetened water every night up to three months, because the baby used to cry every night, and the doctor at the clinic which the mother attended advised this additional bottle; from three to four months, supplementary bottle-feeds, because the mother was tired.
> Mme. L. weaned the child at four months, because of her fatigue, and because she thought four months of mother's milk sufficient. There was no difficulty in weaning.

197

First thickened feeds at four to five months, taken very easily from the bottle, but refused from a spoon towards seven to eight months. Mme. L. insisted.

Alain was a very hungry baby, and Mme. L. gave him breast or the bottle whenever he woke up and cried. She followed the timetable imposed by the baby himself, otherwise he vomited. This went on until he was eight months old.

He was swaddled during the day up to three to four months; at night up to seven months.

First smile: at one and a half months.

First tooth: at seven months (he now has ten teeth).

Could sit up at eight to nine months, but did not want to sit and Mme. L. used to prop him up with pillows.

Walked at fifteen months.

First words: eight months ('papa', 'mama', 'listen').

Present weight: 10·750 kg. ; length: 76 cm.

Alain and his sister are bathed every morning in a large basin, but he has a baby's bath which is used during the summer.

At present he has four meals: a bottle in the morning, which he takes hungrily. At midday he sits at the table with his parents and has the same food as they, just as he does in the evenings. Eats quickly and cleanly. At four o'clock he has yoghourt and plain cakes; but does not take the milk very easily. After he goes to bed in the evening he has another bottle, the last to be kept up of his original feeds.

There is no difficulty with Alain's feeding. He is greedy and likes whatever he is given. Mme. L. never insists if he refuses anything, and does not worry, as his appetite is generally good.

Cleanliness: He was put on the pot at two months; this was the mother's own idea. Mme. L.'s mother lets her please herself about the children, and, on principle, does not give her advice. Mme. L. would hold him out for about a quarter of an hour, then would get tired of it if he had not evacuated. Now, he cries if she insists, but he likes to stay on the pot and play. She lets him do this. Sometimes he does his duty then, but more often afterwards. She scolds him a little: she would very much like him to be clean, as several of her friends' children, of the same age, are so already. It seems that Alain has always been a bit peevish, but Mme. L. notices that he often stamps his foot or whines when she insists on putting him on the pot. She puts him on it just the same.

He urinates in the pot if his mother gets it there in time. She puts him on it regularly, but often he does it on the floor. She then shows him his urine, and scolds him a little 'to make him understand'.

He is very lively, moving about, and walking round the room holding on to the walls and furniture. He bumps into things and falls down, but plays with everything, and prefers objects to games. He plays happily by himself, but has frequent outbursts of temper; he likes to have his own way, says 'no' to everything. When his father is there he gives him a little smack, and prevents him from climbing on to everything. He would be more strict than Mme. L. who prefers peace. Mme. L. lets him cry and he soon stops and comes to make it up. He is affectionate.

Alain often grouses, and cries for no apparent reason. His mother lets him do it, and does not get impatient. He stops when he is given something to play with. He laughs just as readily, and she often plays with him.

Alain is a big, fair baby, and takes after his mother; he is good-natured and smiling. He amused himself quite happily during our visits. Most of all, he needs more room. He is very intelligent and prattles endlessly. He is more frightened of his father than of his mother, who is less strict, more patient, and understanding.

He is left-handed, and Mme. L. does not try to change this. He is very fond of his maternal grandparents, whom he often visits at their home, sometimes staying the night there when his parents are going out for the evening. He does not mind this in the least. He plays with his three-year-old aunt, and pays no attention when his parents leave. Mme. L.'s mother says she does not feel like his grandmother, as she herself has such a young child. He is only frightened when he finds himself alone in a room, which obviously never happens when he is in his own home.

When his sister was born he stayed with his grandmother, and often used to ask for his mother, whom he seemed to miss. They talked to him about a little sister, and he showed great delight on his mother's return.

He has always been very kind to his sister, and his mother has not noticed any change in his attitude since Monique's birth. When his mother changes the baby, he comes too, and watches, kisses the baby, and seems to be very happy. It is the same when the baby is being fed; he has never wanted particularly to get close to his mother at these times, nor become angry. He has always tended to grouse, but this has not got worse since his sister's birth.

Monique

Born after full-term pregnancy, 16th December, 1951, at 'Le Nid' Maternity hospital, at Courbevoie.

> Pregnancy: the mother's condition was good, but the pregnancy was not wanted. She vomited frequently in the first three months.

Confinement: normal;

Weight: 3 kg. Cried immediately.

Breast-feeding supplemented: three bottles and three breast-feeds. Mme. L. had not much milk and this régime was advised in order to avoid tiring her too much. She gives the bottle or the breast (the baby accepts either equally well) when she cries on waking, which is usually at about three-hourly intervals. The baby is very good. She sleeps, feeds, sleeps, feeds . . . She is beginning to smile.

The baby is swaddled, but the clothes are left open at the bottom. She will be swaddled all the winter, but will be dressed in a diaper and little pinafore as soon as the warm weather comes.

Mme. L. will not put her on the pot at two months, as she did with Alain, as she thinks it was a little too early. She will begin at about eight months.

Mme. L. takes her children regularly to the clinic, the baby every week and the elder child every fortnight. They are gaining weight steadily.

At present Mme. L. has no difficulty in rearing her children whom she finds easy to look after, and although she realizes that later on she will have more to worry about, she looks forward to this quite calmly. She considers that she was well brought-up, and will follow more or less the same methods, of freedom, and trust. She will ask for advice from her mother or her mother-in-law if some difficulty should arise; and will be supported, in bringing up her children, by her husband, who, while leaving the main role to her, will always be ready to take his share, as more of a disciplinarian.

The family takes a holiday every year, usually staying with Mme. L.'s grandparents; but now, with two children, they will try to go to the seaside with M. L.'s parents, in a rented villa.

*   *   *   *   *

M. and Mme. L. are a very pleasant young couple, remarkably mature and steady for their age; she is not yet twenty, and he is twenty-three.

It is noteworthy that Mme. L. has overcome various difficulties in her life, such as her father's absence for the five years of the war, while she was still a child of eight to thirteen years of age; the contact with luxury during her apprenticeship in a large Paris fashion house; not to mention the birth of two children within a very short time when she was still very young; the inadequacy of their living conditions, and their dependence on the husband's earnings.

At the same time, the husband, having found himself with family responsibilities while still very young, accepts them cheerfully and with the vigour that he showed when he became a parachutist at eighteen, and that lets him keep up his active interest in sports, without neglecting his family.

EXAMINATION OF DEVELOPMENT

Dr. Marcelle Geber

Alain L. Born 12*th November,* 1950.
Examined 12*th February,* 1952 (15 *months old*).

The test was carried out in the family's only room.

It is a small room of which the whole width is taken up by the parents' bed, while the length just allows for a modern wardrobe to stand by the bed, with a window and the sink alongside. The sink is in a recess, by the side of the gas stove. In front of the wardrobe stands the cot belonging to the little girl of three months. There are also a small table (1·50 m.) and two chairs. The room is very well kept.

Mme. L. is young, slim, pretty, smart.

Alain was lying on his parents' bed, and the little girl was in her cot.

Mme. L. received us in a very friendly way. She said that her main trouble is the smallness of the flat (she has to fold Alain's bed away). But she is hoping to find another one, and meantime puts up with the present conditions, adapting herself to them and managing very well. She replied simply and cordially to questions about her children.

Alain, whom she picked up from the big bed, was at first a bit 'put out'.

Appearance

Alain is a sturdy little boy, and looks very well. He has chubby cheeks, his skin is clear, his expression wide-awake, his hair thick and silky.

His mother sat him on a chair at the small table. He grumbled, and did not want to stay there; and kept turning to his mother, refusing to look at the strange grown-up. But, as soon as he was given some blocks, he looked at them, turned again to his mother, and then his face brightened, and he seemed to be quite at ease.

His mother told us that today he had not had his usual afternoon sleep.

TEST

Alain began the test about five minutes after being sat up for this purpose.

He began by looking at the cubes with interest, then, copying me, tried to build a tower.

He then accepted normally the succession of different objects used in the test, being equally interested in all of them.

He began to chatter, particularly when he was given the book. He picked out the pictures, laughed, was quite at his ease.

When he was given the ball, he threw it to the ground, then got down to look for it and played with it by himself.

He did not protest or cry when the last test item was taken from him. He watched it being put away, then he went towards the bed on which he was lying when we came in. He accepted the medical examination very well.

The test was uniform, the result of good quality, corresponding in level to that of a higher age than that of this child.

It lasted 20 minutes.

(1) *Development*

(a) *Motor*

Locomotor Development: took his first steps several days previously. He sets off, stops, collapses on to the floor, picks himself up. He climbs the stairs on all fours. He can seat himself on a child's little chair and climb on to an adult chair.

He is quite happy, and sure of himself.

At fifteen months his development corresponds to that of sixteen months: L.Q. = 105

Manual dexterity: his movements are neat and precise.

His prehension is good, he grasped the cubes, took the lozenge between the index finger and the thumb, turned the pages of the book two to three at a time.

He is left-handed.

His manual dexterity is clearly superior: eighteen months—M.D.Q. = 118.

(b) *Adaptivity*

He is rapidly adapting his neuro-muscular development to the execution of certain actions, and it was with great precision and accuracy that he took hold of the lozenge to put it into the bottle, then turned the latter upside down to get the lozenge out again; that he made the two-storey tower, set in place the round block, and piled the blocks on top; that he scribbled.

Here, again, he is advanced: seventeen and a half months. A.Q. = 115.

(c) *Language*

Expression: He talks readily, chattering, laughing, pronouncing four or five words correctly, naming the ball.

His ability to express himself is that of a child of sixteen and a half months. E.Q. = 108.

Comprehension: He looks at pictures, fondles them, picks them out.

His comprehension corresponds to sixteen months. C.Q. = 105.

(d) *Personal-Social*

Alain feeds himself, not very cleanly. Toilet-training is not yet complete; he is able to indicate when his knickers are wet. He likes to play, offers a toy, or throws it away when he does not want it. He can make himself understood when he wants something. He pulls along a toy car. However, it is in this sphere that his progress is the least marked: fifteen and a half months. P.S.Q. = 101.

(2) *Behaviour*

(1) *When faced with a new situation:*

He did not accept the strangers immediately, but looked at the toys without picking them up, turned to his mother, a little peevish; then suddenly became interested and accepted the situation.

(2) *With objects:*

After hesitating for a few moments, although looking with interest at the objects, he began to handle them. After that, he showed interest in every object, did each test actively, laughed, chattered and seemed to be well pleased.

(3) *When meeting a strange adult:*

He did not accept her spontaneously. The tester had to speak gently to him, cajole him with toys. But when once he got confidence, he used her extensively, looking at her, talking, laughing, giving her things, taking them back from her, touching her to show her something.

(4) *In relation to his mother:*

Appearing at first to be frightened of this strange adult, he turned to his mother. Then, when he had gained confidence, he just looked at his mother from time to time to assure himself that she was still there.

(3) *The Mother*

Shared the child's activities, watching him and answering if he asked questions. She reassured him gently and softly at the beginning, when he seemed to be frightened of the stranger. She smiled at him, but left him alone, interesting herself in the test, but leaving the examiner to deal with the child.

Conclusion

The physical appearance and wide-awake expression are those of a bright, healthy child.

His development is superior to that of a child of his age: DQ = 108. He is evenly developed, with a more marked advance in manual dexterity and adaptability.

His behaviour is that of a happy and satisfied child, showing interest in everything, and, after a little hesitation, accepting and using the strange adult a great deal.

The mother's attitude contributes to this harmonious development and satisfactory behaviour, as she is herself healthy, balanced and cheerful.

PHYSICAL EXAMINATION

Dr. Cyrille Koupernik

Alain L. Born 12th November, 1950.
Examined 18th February, 1952, at the age of 15 months.

Previous History

Alain is the first-born. It was the mother's first pregnancy; she was 19 years old.

The pregnancy was uneventful; foetal movements were less noticeable than those of his sister, who is now two months old.

He was born at full term; the confinement took place at the local hospital. His weight at birth was 3·100 kg. (6lb. 10oz.)

Labour lasted eighteen hours. No anaesthetic or analgesics. Partial breech presentation; no forceps. He cried immediately; no cyanosis at birth.

During the first days of his life he had neither cyanosis nor icterus. He was very hungry and had no trouble with either suction or swallowing.

During the first months:

He was a rather placid baby, ready to sleep during the day, but crying every night. For this the doctor at the clinic advised the giving of a bottle of sweetened water during the first months.

He smiled at his mother at one and a half months; ocular pursuit was established at about two months.

Head control was a little late (exact date not known).

Could sit up without support at about nine–ten months, could stand at about twelve months, could walk holding on to something at about thirteen months; had just taken his first steps alone (fifteen months).

The mother estimates that spontaneous prehension appeared at about seven–eight months.

First tooth at seven months (he has ten at present).

There has never been any trouble about feeding; he had his first thickened feed at six months, and his first purée at eight months.

Toilet-training was started at two months. Since the age of ten months his mother has been able to tell when he is going to have a rectal evacuation, morning and evening. For some days he had been putting his hand to his pants when he wished to urinate; he does not express his wish in words.

First word: 'papa', at seven–eight months. Has 'talked' since he was eleven–twelve months, and began to understand words at about one year. At present says about five words.

History of Previous Illnesses: Alain was born with a bilateral hydrocele, which was entirely palpable; and a right inguinal hernia, but he was not made to wear a bandage for this. He has had no infectious illness, no otitis, no diarrhoea. No signs of epileptic fits, no screaming attacks.

Vaccinated against smallpox, successfully, at four months, without any general reaction.

There is no significant history of illness in his parents, or their forebears.

He has a sister of two months, who is healthy.

Present Condition

Alain is a fine chubby-faced child, with pink cheeks and firm flesh, and well-coloured mucous membranes.

He weighed, at the time of examination, 10·750 kg. (22¼ lb.).
His length is 0·76 m. (30 in.).

His head circumference is 46 cm. (20 in.).

He stands upright clinging on to the furniture, but is able to keep his balance without support. His walking is still unsteady, with short quick steps; he throws out his feet considerably when walking.

His manual dexterity is good; he has a tendency to use his left hand (his maternal grandmother is left-handed).

Play: He knows how to '*faire les marionnettes*' when asked. His play is still rather motor in type: he likes to bang and throw things; he does not play much, as yet, with dolls and woolly animals; he likes to pull a little toy car along, and to turn the pages of a book.

Comprehension and language: Alain understands simple sentences, such as: 'Where is papa?', 'Where is your little sister?', 'We are going out'.

He knows the use of daily objects, such as spoon and pencil.

He talks baby-talk fluently, and can say about five words: 'Mama, no, wait, bow-wow, bye-bye'.

He does not say when he wants to urinate; he cries when he is hungry.

He likes looking at himself in the mirror, and laughs; he does not appear to recognize himself yet.

Behaviour: He sleeps in his parents' room (the only room in the apartment).

He is not afraid of the dark.

He loves dogs.

He burnt himself once, and since then has been frightened of the stove.

He is not frightened of space, or of water.

He was very frightened recently when he saw his maternal grandfather dressed to go fishing.

He takes his food readily, with enjoyment; he does not have to be coaxed or amused at meal-times. He is very fond of meat and of yoghourt.

He still has a bottle in the evening, which helps him to get to sleep.

He gets into a temper if he is thwarted; he stamps his foot, but he does not roll on the floor, no breath-holding.

On the whole, he is very cheerful, laughs easily.

He is beginning to be a little shy with strangers.

He is equally fond of his father and mother, and has no preference for either men or women. He adores children.

He has not, up to now, shown any jealousy of his little sister, aged 2 months.

He does not suck his thumb. During the first year he used to bang his head against the sides of his cot.

206

Neurological examination:

Shows no sign of abnormality.

Alain has a good standing and sitting posture. There is evidence merely of a slackness of the right muscles of the right side of the abdomen on passive movement from a lying down position to a sitting position.

He has a right inguinal hernia, the size of a pigeon's egg, not descending into the scrotum.

In short, he has a general normal hypotonus common to his age. The joints of the lower limbs are hyper-extensible; in particular, he can do the splits (passively). There is no significant difference of tone between the two sides.

The patellar and the achilles tendon reflexes and the radial reflexes are normal and equal on each side.

The plantar skin reflex is bilaterally flexor.

There are no signs of rickets.

3. THE C. FAMILY
(*Urban Working-Class*)

Mme. Laurette Amado

The family consists of the father, aged 33 years 6 months; the mother, aged 30, and their four children:—Jacqueline 5½ years old; Roger 3½ years old; André 23 months old; Eliane 2 months old.

They live in Paris in a working-class street of the 5th Arrondissement, on the second floor of a very mean dwelling. They have one room and a tiny kitchen.

The water is on the staircase, between the first and second floors. W.C.s for the whole house are in the courtyard. There are gas and electricity. The lighting in the room is indirect, from sconces on the walls. The room is medium-sized, red-tiled. A divan, folded up by day, is the parents' bed. A sideboard contains the children's beds. There is a cot for the baby, Eliane; and a white folding kitchen-table, covered with linoleum.

The rest of the furniture consists of a wardrobe with a mirror; four chairs; and a little low table, with a large photograph of the children, and a vase of flowers. A wireless set stands on the combined sideboard-bed. At night the children's and parents' beds are let down and there is no more space in the room. If you want to move you have to climb over the beds.

The front door leads straight into this room, which has no window, and is therefore only lighted by the little window in the kitchen and the electric light, which is on practically the whole day.

The kitchen, a small room to the left of the bedroom, is hardly separated from it. There is the space for a non-existent door, and the dividing wall has only been built up to about 50 centimetres. You therefore see all the kitchen from the bedroom, which is lighted by the former. (It is evidently on account of the lighting question that the partition has not been built.) The kitchen is very small and crowded. There is a large stove, sideboard and table, with saucepans, vegetables and milk bottles everywhere. It is very difficult to be tidy in such a small room, with six people. Monsieur C.'s bicycle is kept there; he only uses it in the summer.

There is an aquarium on the dividing wall. A small sky-light also lets in a little light to the kitchen. This flat is admitted to be unhealthy. It is very damp.

208

Monsieur and Madame C. have lived there since their marriage, and are still waiting for a city council flat. They are greatly inconvenienced by this situation, but are patient about it.

Madame C.

Born in Paris in the 14th Arrondissement, 12th April, 1922. An only daughter of divorced parents.

Her mother: Aged 48, has been employed for several years in a pharmacy, where her work is valued. She is considered 'odd'. She is very self-centred, not domesticated and never has been, she never bothered about her daughter whom she often reproached for having been born. She has always lived in lodgings and her daughter got in her way. She is very independent, very gay, 'perhaps too much so', said Madame C. She does not want to grow old, and acts all the time, threatening suicide, even now, with her daughter; she is very selfish and disobliging.

She is not affectionate, even with her grandchildren, except the eldest, which annoys Madame C. who does not like favouritism with children.

Her father: Aged 52, was a jewel setter before the war, in a good situation, but his tools were destroyed in the war, and he has not been able to replace them owing to the high cost. He is living now in the suburbs with his mother and a brother. He gardens and does odd jobs, and is very understanding, kind, cheerful, serious and affectionate. He has never spoken against his wife to his daughter, and has not married again.

Her stepfather: Aged 46, a store-keeper in a cork factory. He has always been kind to his step-daughter, gives her presents, and is much more affectionate than his wife. He has been in bad health ever since his return from captivity, in 1945.

Madame C. was at first put out to nurse in the Chevreuse Valley. She was never breast-fed. When she was born her father was doing his military service, and her mother did not want to keep her, preferring her freedom. She was very badly cared-for when out at nurse, and was very ill when twenty months old. The foster-mother warned the family, and in this way the maternal grandparents, at whose house the letter arrived, learnt of the existence of their granddaughter. Very annoyed at the attitude of their daughter, they made her go and fetch the child immediately, for they wanted to keep the child at their home in the Yonne department.

There Madame C. was very well looked after, the grandparents being very kind and affectionate. They were small-holders on their own account. They kept their grandchild until she was thirteen. She thrived, and was in very good health, gave no trouble, and was devoted to them. She used to see her parents two or three times a year.

The latter had separated when Madame C. was three and a half years old, and divorced when she was nine, in 1931. From this time on, each saw their daughter separately, and she practically never saw them together. They had never got on well together, although they did not quarrel; but Madame C.'s mother had always been very independent, not bothering about daughter or husband. She left her husband for a lover, then for another, who became her second husband in 1935.

Madame C., when five and a half, had the experience of being abandoned by her mother, who had come to stay with her parents, where her daughter was living. One day when she was out walking with her, Madame C. heard a whistle, and saw a shadow; and her mother then asked her to go and fetch her scarf from the house, as she was cold. The child refused, having a foreboding that if she left her mother she would never see her again. Her mother insisted, so she went, and when she returned, her mother had gone. She quickly warned her grandmother, who told the father; he came next morning, and after police investigations, they traced the fugitive, with her lover, to an hotel.

Madame C. remembers this scene well. She felt that her mother did not love her, since she could leave her for a man who was not her father. She thinks maternal love should have prevailed.

A little later, her father, an aunt, an uncle and Madame C. went to find her mother in the lodgings where she was living with her lover, to try to persuade her to return home. She refused; then seems to have returned for a week, and gone away again. Madame C. has never forgiven her mother; she says she loves her from a sense of duty.

Madame C. went to school, and worked well: but she did not take her Certificate of Primary Education, for at this time her mother took her back to Paris to put her to work. According to the divorce decree, she had no right to do this, as the guardianship of the child was given to the grandparents. But they and the father did not wish to make trouble, and allowed her to do as she wished. Madame C. was taken on in a laboratory where, so she said, she worked as assistant chemist till the age of eighteen. She lived with her mother and stepfather in a flat of three rooms and a kitchen. Madame C. had her own room.

She gave them all her money, and got on quite well, for they each went their own way; but the mother's lack of affection and selfishness did not encourage closer ties between her and her daughter.

Then came the war. Her stepfather was mobilized, and her mother, frightened of the bombing, for two years took refuge with her daughter at her parents' home in the Yonne department. She did not work and did not feel well. Madame C. helped her grandmother in the fields and in the house.

In 1942, mother and daughter returned to Paris. Madame C. was taken on at the cork factory where her stepfather worked, but she had to leave, because of advances made by her employer. Then she went into a stylo-pen factory where she remained till her marriage, in October, 1945. Her husband was a childhood friend. The maternal grandmothers of both were friends, and Madame C. had always known her husband. They saw each other in their families in childhood, and when about sixteen or seventeen years old, became engaged. The families knew about the plan, but considered they were too young to marry; especially as at this time Madame C.'s mother had other young men in view for her daughter, but she would have none of them.

Throughout the war, Madame C. remained faithful to this young man and after his return from captivity they were married. She loved him very much, respected him and thought him very serious-minded and stable. She seems to understand him well.

Madame C. is a fat, chubby little woman, talkative and full of life. She is rather untidy in her dress, putting her children's needs before her own with regard to clothes. She was wearing a pleated tartan skirt, blue pull-over, apron, rope shoes, no stockings. She wears no make-up at all, but has a high colour. She has a pleasant face, and seems in perfect health. She has never been ill, except for diphtheria two years ago. She began to menstruate at thirteen, and did not know what it was. She told a seventeen-year-old boy friend that she was 'wounded' and was bleeding, and when he wanted to see where, in order to care for the wound, she refused. He then realised what it was, and advised her to put on a towel. She dared not say anything to her grandmother, who became aware of it the next day on seeing the stained sheets. She then said to her 'Now you're a big girl, you mustn't talk to little boys', so at school she no longer spoke to the boys.

She had had no sexual education before she worked in the factory after the war. There, her companions talked coarsely, and she learned a good deal, but it was her husband who initiated her, with great tact, she said. She gets on very well with him, fortunately, for he is a particular man on this subject and wants his wife to be responsive.

Madame C. does not intend to leave her children in ignorance, as she was, and will explain these things to them. She considers that this should be done by the mother.

She is intelligent. Now and again she shows a little vanity; her husband evidently considers her more intelligent than himself, better informed and able to discuss things. She said she had read a good deal during the time she was living with her mother in Paris. She joined a library and read everything—novels, poetry, and particularly medical books, from which she learnt about conception, birth, etc. She used to go to the cinema and theatre with her mother and stepfather, but her husband has never had this 'Parisian' life.

Madame C. is much attached to her children; she is very motherly, affectionate and gentle with them. She appears to bring them up by combining authority and affection, and playing on the latter in order to get obedience. She pretends to cry, or threatens to go away, if they do not obey; and at once they are obedient; but she only uses this method as a last resort.

She is patient and calm, never loses her temper. She is cheerful, trusting and very talkative, and received us with great kindness, confidence and simplicity, taking our interview in good part. She speaks quickly, loudly, with a slight lisp.

She was affectionate with the children during our visits, and seemed to look after them with great tenderness. She is very lively and active, gets up at 4.30 a.m., to work while her children sleep. Nearly all her afternoons are free to take the children out.

Madame C.'s maternal grandparents are dead. *Her grandmother* died in 1945, aged 74, of congestion of the lungs. She was a woman of splendid robust health, who used to work on the land. Very affectionate and cheerful, she took excellent care of her granddaughter till her thirteenth year. She used to say she 'was the most beautiful flower in her garden'. She was not stern, shouted sometimes, but never struck her. She never, in front of her granddaughter, criticized her daughter's behaviour although she felt it keenly.

Her grandfather died in 1932, aged 65, as a result of an accident at work. They were smallholders, but he used to work in a saw-mill as well. He was very good, calm, a cheerful companion. Madame C. was deeply attached to these grandparents, far more so than to her father's parents, whom she had hardly known.

Monsieur C.

Born on 13th July, 1918, in the Yonne department. He never knew his father, and his mother was unmarried at the time of his birth. Monsieur C. had a difficult childhood.

His mother: Aged 57, lives in Rheims where she has had a post in a family for five years. There are five children, and she is looked on as one of the family.

She is well disposed, though somewhat difficult and not very understanding. Above all, she is weak, and needs a man, not knowing how to get along alone. She is unstable and unreliable, yet she is kind and a good sort; she loved her eldest son as a matter of pride.

His father was either killed or disappeared during the 1914 war. Monsieur C.'s mother was engaged to him, and became pregnant after his last leave, since when she had no further news of him. He seems to have been handsome and attractive. She had some difficulty with her family on account of the pregnancy before marriage.

Monsieur C.'s mother set up house with another man, and brought up her child, not going out to work. Monsieur C. remembered this time when, up to the age of six years, he was happy with his mother.

Later, his mother went out to work, and from then on he was unhappy, left to himself all day and not being able to eat when he was hungry. He says that often for three days on end neither he nor his parents had a morsel of bread. He wonders what could have become of the money earned by both. This mystery was not even solved by his mother, to whom he spoke about it recently. She had said to him, weeping, 'that she had not had the money to buy food for him'. His wife said to us afterwards that certainly at that time her mother-in-law had another lover (the first was ill in hospital), and not daring to bring him to the house, she often used to go to him.

At this time his mother did not look after him at all, and he feels this keenly and also the possibility that he might have reacted strongly to this treatment. But not wanting to let himself go, he bottled it all up inside himself. He never seems to have had any character problems. This painful time, which he recalls with emotion, ended at the age of eight, when he entered the Rheims Children's Home where he remained till he was thirteen. They were the best years of his childhood. The people who looked after the seventy children there were decent women, who loved them as though they were their own. The house was well run, the food plentiful, and Monsieur C. has really pleasant memories of it. He attended the local primary school and worked well.

In the summer holidays he used to spend a month with his mother, who was then re-married to a Portuguese, a jolly fellow, strong, and kind, with whom he got on well. This stepfather, now about forty-five years old, could not own him at the time of the marriage because there was not enough difference in their ages, only eleven or twelve years. Monsieur C. therefore bears his mother's maiden name. The stepfather was employed by a wine business (Caves Remoises), and he earned good wages. They built a house for themselves with three rooms in addition to a kitchen and dining-room. The house was surrounded by a garden. Six children were born of this marriage. They all live in Rheims.

The parents have been divorced since the war, at the beginning of which Madame C. kindly took in a sick friend younger than herself. The husband subsequently left home with this woman, and this led to a divorce. Monsieur C.'s mother was very much upset by this fresh blow. Now she is at work, as her children are no longer dependent on her, the two youngest living with the father and the others married. When Monsieur C. returned from Germany he found his parents already separated and their house sold. He has never known much about this period. He never had any close relationship with his half-brothers and sisters, but was never on bad terms with them.

At the age of thirteen, just as he was going to pass his Certificate of Primary Education, his mother took him away from the Children's Home as she wished him to work. He very much regrets never having obtained this diploma. Until he was eighteen he worked in a chocolate factory in Rheims. Then he joined the infantry, in 1938, and went to the war; he was taken prisoner and sent to Germany until May, 1945.

It was a very active period for Monsieur C. He was a 'dare-devil' and always headstrong; he wanted to join the 'Free Corps'. It was a time of adventure which he enjoyed, but army life did not really appeal to him. He was very serious-minded, as he had always been. During his captivity he was a ringleader in his camp, and tried to ensure that the prisoners would not give way to discouragement and depression. He organized theatrical shows in the camp.

In military life he was looked upon as a dandy, for he was always well-groomed; he used to shave, wash his clothes etc., at a time when others let themselves go. But he was always well thought of by his superiors, without his ever having sought favour. While a prisoner he worked practically all the time, which ensured his being better fed. He did not have too many difficulties on his return home.

In the camps in Germany, the prisoners used to talk of French women without much respect. Germans returning from France brought back stories and photographs which did not give them a high opinion of many French women, to such an extent that on his return he did not think of marrying. He wished to enjoy life for at least five years. However, Monsieur C. came back via Paris, knowing that there he would see his childhood friend. He was very fond of her, had photographs of her, but during his captivity he had had no news of her, and had not thought of her as a possible wife. He was pleased to meet her again, and on his second visit his future mother-in-law told him that her daughter was still waiting for him. He therefore decided to marry, although he had not thought of it previously, and was very pleased with this development.

As to work, he was taken on, in 1945, at a large car factory, where

214

he is still working on the production line. It is quick work, paid as 'piece work'; he works overtime 'for the children'—58 hours a week. He earns more than 50,000 frs. a month, plus family allowances. He reckons it is good pay which he would not easily find elsewhere, and for that reason remains there.

The factory is far from his home. He leaves at 6 a.m., and returns at 6.30 p.m. and has only half an hour for lunch, which he does not have in the canteen, but takes with him. In summer he bicycles to work.

We saw Monsieur C. on his return from the factory. Tall, slight, very well groomed. He wore a blue suit in excellent taste, with a tie and scarf. He tidies himself at the factory every evening. He is reticent, but his somewhat distant manner is due to shyness and an inferiority complex, and also to his rather rigid temperament. He is suspicious and timid; these are the defences he has used from his earliest years; but beneath this he is very kind, gentle, calm, serious, frank, courageous, well-balanced, the very opposite of his mother, Madame C. tells us.

He is intelligent, and regrets not having taken his Certificate of Primary Education. He thinks he does not know how to express himself, and says he talks little because he fears the conversation will lead on to a level where he will no longer be able to follow—theatre, books, etc.—and also because he thinks that people talk a great deal, and say nothing. He prefers silence to the endless, dull gossip in which many people pass their time.

He was very pleased with his conversation with us. We found that he expressed himself fluently and well. He was most agreeable and confiding. Although he says he is cheerful, he has a sad look. Nevertheless he is neither disillusioned nor bitter. One feels that he has lived through difficult moments, to which he has reacted by shutting himself off from the outward world, never losing grip of himself, and always wishing to remain master of himself.

He is very fond of children, and could ill have borne not to have had any. He is very pleased with his little family. In the evening they are all over him with their play; he is very kind and patient with them. Above all he wishes them not to be unhappy, as he was. He does not like to be separated from them, and immediately regrets their absence. He is, however, quite strict with them, and when told to do a thing, he expects them to obey. He succeeds in this better than his wife.

He likes order and cleanliness, and certainly suffers more than his wife from the smallness of their flat and the disorder in the kitchen. He disapproves of a certain slipshodness in his wife, who for instance, goes out in rope shoes, or an apron, when she could quite well put on her shoes. He is certainly punctilious in all these matters, but is evidently able to control himself and not make violent objections, for he never quarrels with his wife.

Monsieur C. is very jealous, will not let himself be made a fool of, and does not like having men friends at the house. He talks very little even in the family circle, though his wife says that some evenings he begins to talk and will go on all through the night.

Monsieur C. is in very good health and has never been ill. Before the war he went in for sport (boxing and swimming). His wife made him give up boxing as she did not want him to be disfigured. He no longer has time for sport, and contents himself with fishing. In the evening on returning from the factory he is tired and does not want to read anything but the sporting paper. For some time he has had trouble with his eyes. He likes cooking and does it well, and often on Sunday he prepares the dinner. He is a handyman, but does not like housework. Besides, his wife would not want him to do it, and manages so that all is done in time for his return. He does not drink, and smokes only a little.

Monsieur and Madame C. make a happy home. They are certainly linked by their difficult childhood, and their affection for their children. They have few hobbies in common. However, on Saturday evenings they often arrange for the children to be looked after by a woman, whom they pay, and they go to the cinema. On Sundays in the summer they go fishing in the ponds, near Paris, rented by Monsieur C.'s factory for their workpeople. They picnic and are very happy.

On Sundays they are also often visited by Madame C.'s mother and her husband. This does not altogether please Madame C. as her mother is thoughtless and tactless, talking of the 'matches' her daughter might have made, threatening suicide, etc.

The budget is managed by Madame C., to whom her husband regularly hands over his pay. She hands back to him 2,000 or 3,000 frs. for pocket money, in addition to money for his fares and canteen, but he does not spend the money, and out of it buys presents for his wife and children. He is going to buy a chiming clock for their new flat.

Madame C. does not keep account of expenses, and has practically no difficulties over money. They are saving up in order to furnish the flat they hope to have soon. They listen to the wireless, and Madame C. reads women's magazines lent to her by friends in the house.

She belongs to a Mothers' Club in her district, where 'trained' workers, a social worker, and the mothers talk about the children, ask advice, etc.

Monsieur and Madame C. are Catholics, and practised their religion till Jacqueline's birth. Throughout his life, and especially in captivity, religion has greatly helped Monsieur C.

Jacqueline

Born at eight and a half months, on 5th July, 1946, in a Parisian maternity hospital. Madame C. and her husband both wanted their first child to be a girl: 'Girls soon help their mother'. No sickness, pregnancy very well borne, but some difficulty at the moment of birth as Madame C. has a narrow pelvic cavity (injections of post-pituitrin and quinine). However, delivery was normal; child cried immediately; weight 3·950 kg.

Breast-fed entirely till thirteenth month. Madame C. always has plenty of milk and wants to feed her babies as long as possible. She thinks it is better for them.

Six feeds a day, never at night, gave her the breast when she awoke, at roughly three-hour intervals. She fed the child as long as she wanted it.

First thickened feed: at thirteen months, from a spoon. Has never had a bottle.
First smile: at one month.
First tooth: at four and a half months.
First word: at seven months.
First sentences: at fifteen months; speaks very well.
Walked: at one year.
Wore swaddling clothes by day till two months old; by night, till ten months old.
Cleanliness: at nine months (?) by day; at two years, by night.

She was put on the pot from the age of four months, and made use of it about every other time. She sleeps well, has a very good appetite, is always hungry. Madame C. has never had any difficulty with Jacqueline about food. No sucking habits. Jacqueline is a pretty little dark-haired girl, dainty, with a bright complexion. She is slender and not very big for her age, very good-tempered and quiet, a coquette, who knows exactly what she wants. She might be rather self-willed, but not ill-tempered. Very affectionate and devoted to her father. Before the birth of her last little sister, she used to say 'Papa and I have ordered a little sister'. She is merry, not jealous or grumpy. She plays a great deal with her brothers and sister, especially at 'Papa and Mama' (she is the mother).

She is beginning to help her mother a bit, clears the table, and looks after her brother. 'She is an argumentative little Miss' said her mother. Every morning and afternoon she goes to the kindergarten with her brother Roger. She always has the Croix d'Honneur (good conduct mark).

She has never been ill, except for German measles in 1948. She has never asked any questions about her mother's pregnancies, and has always welcomed her brothers and sister.

Roger

Born on 11th June, 1948, at full term, at the Maternity Hospital. Pregnancy was easy, never ill or tired. Mme. C. and her husband both wanted a boy.

Normal birth. Weight 4.300 kg.; cried immediately. Breast-fed till sixteen months, six feeds, as for Jacqueline.

First thickened feed: at thirteen months.

First smile: at one month.

First tooth: at six months.

First words: at eight months.

First sentences: at fourteen months; has a defect in pronunciation (does not pronounce R).

Walked: at fourteen months.

Good appetite: sleeps well.

Cleanliness: at nine–ten months. Wet his bed till he was put on the pot, from the age of four to five months.

Roger is a plump little fellow, who has no troubles. Everything is always all right. He plays all day, and at night is dropping with sleep. He sings and dances all the time.

He is even more affectionate than his sister. Every morning as soon as he is awake he comes in to find his mother in the kitchen and says 'Good morning, Mother, I love you with all my heart'. He apparently instituted this ceremony himself. He is very coaxing, sensitive, more unreserved and easy-going than his sister. Has no habits, such as using a dummy, etc. Last year he had the beginnings of otitis but except for that, has never been ill. Goes to the kindergarten, where he is very happy.

Roger is indeed 'the jolly, fat boy', fair and smiling, with a nice affectionate manner.

André

Born on 26th April, 1950, at full term, in the same maternity hospital as his sister and brother.

An easy pregnancy, without fatigue. Madame C. was still nursing Roger when she was pregnant. Although another child was not wished for, he was immediately welcomed by his father and mother, who wanted another boy.

Normal birth, shoulder presentation, manipulation to change the position. Weight 4·500 kg. child cried immediately.

Breast-fed up to eighteen months, six feeds a day, never at night. Given the breast when he woke up, until he relinquished it.

First thickened feed: at about one year; well liked.

First smile: at one month.

First tooth: at seven months (now has twenty).

First sat up: at six months.

First words: at six and a half months.

First sentences: at sixteen months.

Walked: at one year.

Wore swaddling clothes till two months old by day, and ten months at night. Has never been ill except for bronchitis this winter, treated with penicillin.

Food. Has always eaten well, with no difficulty at all. Likes everything, is very greedy. At the present time has four meals a day.

Morning: white coffee, or chocolate, with bread and butter.

Midday: soup, vegetables, meat, fruit.

Afternoon: Bread, chocolate or fruit.

Evening: soup, vegetables, fruit.

From the age of one he has fed himself, and has meals with his brother and sister. They eat quickly and early, at 6.30 p.m., before their parents. Madame C. puts them to bed at once and then dines with her husband. At midday she lunches with them. She does not allow the children to speak at table.

Sleep. André sleeps well and soundly from 7 p.m. to 6 a.m. Madame C. puts him back to bed for a little while during the morning for from half to three-quarters of an hour. Since the age of one he has rarely slept in the afternoon, but goes out with his mother. Like the others, he has never cried at night. He sleeps with his teddy-bear, and does not put himself to sleep with a dummy.

Cleanliness. He was put on the pot from the age of four to five months, and was clean from the age of seven months. Madame C. had kept a watch on the time at which he usually evacuated, and from the age of five months put him on his pot at that time. In this way he very quickly got used to not messing himself. Madame C. wanted this early cleanliness, as she did not like leaving the children in their soiled napkins, and feared that delayed cleanliness might be a symptom of illness. From one year old he has asked for, and goes by himself to his 'chair pot', which stays permanently in the kitchen. For the last two months he has been clean at night; he calls for his mother so that she can get him up.

Games. He likes playing, plays with everything, and is not destructive. He has many toys. His own are a bicycle, ball, cubes, etc., and he also plays with those belonging to his brother and sister. He amuses himself happily by himself. Is a bit of a 'dare-devil', and very 'tough' when he falls.

André is obedient, especially with his father. He is gentle, affectionate and loves to be caressed on his mother's knees. Very cheerful, laughs all the time, never grumbles. Has never been jealous, and is always good-tempered. Is very resourceful.

With his little sister he is especially affectionate. He comes and kisses her when she is at the breast, and always wants to be near her, caressing her gently. He never seems to have any aggressive feeling towards her. He does not particularly seek his mother's attention when she is busy with Eliane. There has been no change in his manner since Eliane's birth.

Outings. André goes out several times a day. Morning and evening he goes with his mother to take Jacqueline and Roger to and from school. In the afternoon he goes with his mother to the park. He loves being out of doors.

He is a fair child, with very bright eyes, and a mischievous expression. He is very smiling, restless, climbs everywhere, and tries to make off with sweets. He does not yet speak very well; his language is somewhat incomprehensible for the uninitiated.

He has a dummy in his mouth, attached to a cord round his neck; he did not ask for this dummy, it was his father who put it in his mouth to silence him. He talks incessantly, rather loudly, and his father, at the end of his patience, gave him the dummy. André has not become addicted to it; he does not want it, and does not go to sleep with it. He is ashamed of it, and on our arrival hid it behind a handkerchief.

Eliane

Born on 8th January, 1952, in the Maternity Hospital.

An easy pregnancy, no sickness. The child was not wanted, but was quickly accepted by all the family.

Normal birth, at full term.

Weight: 4·460 kg.; child cried immediately.

Breast-fed: six feeds a day.

First smile: at one month. A fine baby, dimpled and smiling.

As Madame C.'s mother had said that they must not rely on her to look after the children during the confinement, it was the mother-in-law who came to help. She was at first very pleased, but as the birth was delayed, she quickly got impatient and finally was very happy to return to Rheims. Then she wrote that she was annoyed, and now she does not even answer the two weekly letters Madame C. regularly sends her.

Madame C. has never menstruated since her marriage. She was pregnant from the earliest days, and later, with the four births and prolonged feeding, she has never had her periods. She has a great deal of milk, and since André's birth, the third child, she has given some to the hospitals. She can give at least a litre a day. It is called for daily, and she is paid 800 francs a litre.

On the question of the children's upbringing, M. and Mme. C. are in agreement. In principle it is the mother who makes herself responsible, although the father is also interested. He has more authority than she, and the children obey him instantly, whereas Madame C. has to use various devices, such as threats, promises, and even 'blackmail'. But, on the whole, the children are obedient. Madame C. also reasons with them, and does not treat them as 'babies'. To André, who was crying in our presence, she said most affectionately 'You are a man, and a man does not cry like that'. He stopped. She has principles about upbringing. She will not have her children talking slang. She will not allow them to talk at meals; silence is observed.

She is very pleased to send her children to a 'religious' school, where they learn good manners, and on the whole she appreciates the nuns' teaching. This summer Jacqueline will go to a holiday home run by nuns.

The children seem very responsive to their mother's wishes. Roger comes immediately and kisses his mother if she scolds him. He is particularly affected if his mother pretends to cry, or says she will go away.

In principle Madame C. does not smack or slap. She will not beat the children, thinks it is not a good method. Jacqueline, however, receives a slap now and again.

She would rather deprive them of dessert, but when the time comes to give out the fruit, she regrets it, and often cancels the punishment. But she is stricter about sweets. Every evening when their father comes home, there is the 'time for rewards', a kind of collective examination of conscience, presided over by Monsieur C., to whom the children render an account of their good or bad behaviour during the day. Sweets are distributed according to the merits of each one. All this takes place in a happy atmosphere.

Madame C. is very gay, understanding and gentle, and she must have great patience to live with these four children in this unhealthy room, with no conveniences.

221

She is full of fun, and easily comes down to the children's level, knowing how to be an adult at one moment, and at others a child among her children. She is mistress of the situation, and is never overwhelmed, and seems perfectly balanced and in the right place.

Her husband, equally, seems very understanding and gentle, but his more rigid temperament and more tenacity will give him a sterner manner. At the same time he is less compromising.

The children are very much attached to him, for he is only severe when it is necessary, knowing well (because he himself had painfully experienced it) how great is a child's need of affection. But he knows that this does not exclude judicious doses of authority.

To sum up, Monsieur and Madame C. are a couple united by a long childhood friendship and by hardships in youth, which gave both of them a deep love of children. They are linked also by their constant mutual understanding and a disinterested wish to do right. This attractive family seems to us very well balanced and stable, living simply, with a good spirit, in an invigorating atmosphere of gaiety and optimism.

EXAMINATION OF DEVELOPMENT
Dr. Marcelle Geber

André C. Born 26th April, 1950.
Examined March, 1952 (23 months old).

The test took place in the only room, in the presence of the mother and the three other children.

The room was fairly big, and adjoining it was a small kitchen, with no separating door. The interior was clean, neat and tidy.

When we arrived, Madame C. was playing a game in a circle, in the middle of the room, with her three eldest, whilst the youngest slept in her cradle. She is a young woman, spruce, good-natured and straightforward, and apparently happy. She replied simply and concisely to our questions. She was calm and smiling, and spoke gently to the children, who obeyed her fairly well.

Appearance

André is a little fair boy, chubby, alert, interested and of good physique.

He looked at us somewhat apprehensively, and refused to come near me. Whilst I was showing him the cubes, he looked at them, but would not come near. He remained standing by his mother.

We therefore advised his mother to take him on her lap at the table. André immediately accepted the objects and the tester.

222

TEST

He was interested in all the objects, and became absorbed in them, not making use of his mother, on whose knees he was sitting, but rather of the tester, from whom he accepted the toys, and to whom he talked. His interest was constant and concentrated. He was eager, particularly, for the book. He seemed happy in the sequence of the various test items. The test took twenty minutes and gave a reliable result. The two eldest children gathered round André, who took no notice of them, but pushed them away when they wished to take the testing toys.

When the test was finished, he played with the ball, running round the room laughing.

He protested when we put away the objects, but his mother comforted him immediately.

(1) *Development*

His motor, adaptive and personal-social development are above, and his language development is exactly equal to, that of his chronological age.

(*a*) *Motor*

Locomotion: He walks; runs without falling; goes up and down stairs alone. He kicks the ball with his foot. He tries to stand upright on one foot. He is well developed, good muscular tone, steady on his feet, having the movement of a child of twenty-six months. L.Q. $= 113$.

Manual Dexterity: His grasp is good, precise. He can easily make a tower of six or seven blocks, he turns with ease the pages of the book, one by one. He easily grasps the blocks of the form-board. He is right-handed. His manual dexterity is that of twenty-four months: M.D.Q. $= 104$.

(*b*) *Adaptivity*

He likes playing with the blocks and spontaneously builds a tower, afterwards forming them into a train. He easily fits the pieces into the form-board and quickly adapts himself to turning them round the other way. He promptly inserts the square into its socket.

He immediately pulls the ball out of the bottle.

He delights in free scribbling.

His adaptivity is that of a child of twenty-five months, twelve days. A.Q. $= 110$.

(c) Language

> *Expression:* Speaks phrases of three words, explains himself, and chiefly talks about the book, knows more than twenty words.
>
> *Comprehension:* Recognizes three pictures and obeys four orders with the ball.
>
> His language is therefore well developed, and corresponds exactly to his age—twenty-three months:—
> E.Q. = 100, C.Q. = 100.

(d) Personal–Social

> In this field he is decidedly forward. He asks for food, drink, and to urinate. He holds out his cup, he feeds himself from a spoon, does not spill. He asks fairly regularly to do his business.
>
> He imitates his mother, copying her in her domestic tasks. He plays alongside the children who are with him. He pushes along a toy, and steers it correctly.
>
> He describes in words what he does, speaks of himself in the third person, draws someone aside to show him something.
>
> His reactions are therefore at a level of twenty-five and a half months.
> P.S.Q. = 111.

(2) *Behaviour*

His behaviour is that of a healthy child, happy and blooming.

(a) In a new situation:

> When we entered, he was playing with his mother, and we interrupted the game, so he looked at us somewhat fearfully, seeming to ask himself what exactly we were expecting him to do.
>
> Confidence restored, seated on his mother's knee, he became of his own accord interested in the test, and easily accepted the new situation.

(b) Towards an adult stranger:

> Safely seated on his mother's lap, he readily accepted the tester. He spoke and laughed with her, asked for objects from her, and gave them to her.

(c) Towards his mother:

> With his back turned to his mother, he seemed to enjoy the comfort of being on her lap, but did not directly make use of her. He was absorbed and in-

terested in the toys, and included the tester with them.

At the end of the test, quite at home with the tester, he easily did all his motor tests, enabling his mother to talk to the doctor.

(d) *Towards the two elder children* (4 *and* 5 *years old*):

He pushed them away when they came too close, or wished to take the objects from him. But this was merely a protest, completely understood by the older ones.

(3) *The Mother*

Shared the child's activities, watching him, and in the beginning encouraging him. She described his buoyant health and quick intelligence.

Her manner is warm, but not exaggerated.

The elder brother and sister were interested in the toys, and wanted to join in the test. But they accepted with good grace the protests of André, and obeyed their mother when she advised them to leave André alone.

Conclusion

This child's development is entirely satisfactory. His D.Q. = 105, with a marked advance in neuromuscular maturity which he can put at the service of his intelligence. This enables him to be equally in advance in his social reactions.

His behaviour is that of a happy child, well developed, who trusts grown-ups.

His interest is, in fact, very wide-awake and his hesitation, at the beginning, to accept the adult, was justified by our interruption in the middle of his game.

PHYSICAL EXAMINATION

Dr. Cyrille Koupernik

André C. Born on 26th April, 1950.
Examined on 24th March, 1952 (at the age of 23 months).

Previous History

Mother's third pregnancy.

First child, a daughter, 6 years old. Weight 3·950 kg. (8 lb. 11 oz.) at birth, normal.

Second child, a boy, 4 years old. Weight 4·300 kg. (9 lb. 8 oz.) at birth, normal.

Fourth child, a daughter, 2 months old. Weight 4·460 kg. (9 lb. 13 oz.) at birth, normal.

The mother has never had a miscarriage.

Pregnancy:

Maternal condition good; foetal movements, like the others.

Confinement:

In the maternity wing of a Paris hospital. Child was a month over-due.

Weight: 4·500 kg. (9 lb. 14 oz.)

Labour lasted six hours.

The mother was not anaesthetized.

She was given an injection of post-pituitrin.

Vertex presentation.

Cried immediately. No cyanosis at birth.

First days:

No cyanosis, no jaundice.

Some difficulty with sucking.

First development:

The child smiled at a human face at about one month old.

Voluntary grasp at three months.

Early control of head movements.

Sitting position, unsupported, from five to six months old, stand-ing up at eight months, walked by himself at one year.

Toilet-training began at about four to five months.

Bowels—clean at about ten months.

He verbalized his desire to urinate at the age of about fourteen months.

At the present moment he manages his micturition by himself.

He has never had difficulties with appetite.

He began to chew his food at the age of thirteen to fourteen months.

He said his first word ('papa') at six months old, 'mamma' at seven months.

At fourteen months, he verbalized his feeling of hunger.

At twenty-two months he was already saying '*à manger*' ('hun-gry').

He began to understand verbal orders at fourteen months.

At twenty months he said his first phrase.

He began to play with a teddy bear about the age of one year.

From twenty-one months old, he rode a tricycle.

He had his first tooth at seven months.

He has never been ill, except for rhino-pharyngitis at the age of eighteen months.

He has never had convulsions.

He was unsuccessfully vaccinated against smallpox at the age of ten days, and successfully at five months.

He has always been looked after by his mother.

Family History

Mother:	Thirty years old, and healthy.
	Before marriage she worked in a laboratory.
	There is no history of illness in the family.
Father:	Thirty-four years old.
	He is a skilled worker, and healthy.

Generally speaking, the children are more obedient to their father. André is very fond of his little sister, aged two months, and he regards her as his personal property.

Present Behaviour

At the present moment the child runs without much difficulty.

He goes upstairs by himself, step by step; he comes down held by the hand. He climbs on chairs.

He uses his right hand more often than his left, but he is taught to do this.

Games:

He plays with bricks, his teddy bear, and a large ball. He no longer tears up paper.

He rides a tricycle, and is interested in pictures.

He pretends to read the newspaper.

Comprehension and Speech:

He understands practically all the usual words.

He uses a pencil and a spoon by himself.

His vocabulary includes most of the ordinary words. He makes sentences of three words. He calls himself by his Christian name, but at times he says: 'I', and points to himself. When he is in front of a mirror he wants his mother to brush his hair and put eau de Cologne on him.

He recognizes himself in a photograph.

Usual Behaviour:

He sleeps in his parents' room.

He shows no fear.

He manages his food very well, at table with the grown-ups.

He hardly ever gets angry.

He is shy at first with strangers, but quickly gets used to them.

He seems to be equally attached to his father and mother, and makes no difference between men and women.

He likes children very much.

He does not show any jealousy of his little sister, seems very pleased when his mother busies herself with her, and frequently kisses her hands.

Physical Examination

He is a fair child, slightly pale, with blue eyes.

His mucous membranes are well coloured, and his muscles are firm.

> Weight: 12·500 kg. (27½ lb.)
> Height: 84 cm. (2 ft. 9 in.)
> Has 20 teeth.
> Head circumference: 47 cm. (19 in.).

He has an alert and expressive countenance.

His standing position is excellent. He walks without abducting his legs, and his feet rest on the lateral part of the sole. His grasp is normal. He releases objects without difficulty. His movements are precise. He shows a hypotonus, normal for his age, with a slight relaxation of the muscles of the abdomen. The tendon reflexes are normal. His cutaneous plantar reflexes are equivocal. He has phimosis.

Conclusion

A normal child, well adjusted, alert, high-spirited, and not showing problems customary at this age.

Note that he was breast-fed up to eighteen months, practically till the birth of his little sister.

4. THE V. FAMILY
(*Agricultural Workers*)

Mme. Laurette Amado

The V. family consists of the mother, 27 years of age; the father, 28; and their two sons, Aimé, born 9th July, 1947, and Yves, born 19th October, 1950.

They live in an old disused farm-house in the middle of the village. They have two rooms. We only saw the kitchen, which is fairly large, and quite well kept for the country, though it is poor. It is furnished with a large table, a cooking stove, two large sideboards, chairs, many of which are in bad repair, and a sink, made of black stone, though the water supply is in the yard. There is electricity, but only cylinder gas. The kitchen has a sunny aspect, and is on the same level as the yard.

They have an old stable where they put their two goats, the straw, the wood, etc. The W.C. is in the yard.

Madame V.

Born 9th December, 1924, in a neighbouring village.

Her mother: aged 55; is still doing farm work. She is not affectionate, but hard and bad-tempered. She never liked girls, did not want a daughter and made Mme. V.'s life very unhappy during the whole of her childhood.

However, as far as other people are concerned, she is quite pleasant; but Mme. V. speaks of her with a complete lack of affection, and even with bitterness.

Her father: aged 64; a retired road-worker, in very good health, kind; he supported his children.

Eldest brother: aged 28; works in a factory; is married, with two children and a third expected. He lives in the same village as his parents, next door to them.

Second brother: aged 15; is at an apprentice training centre for electricians. Took his C.E.P. (Certificat d'Etudes Primaires); he is kind and affectionate, and comes to see his sister from time to time.

Mme. V. does not see much of her family, nor do they try to have much to do with her. She had not seen her parents for two years, although the villages are only four–five kilometres apart. A few days previously she had decided to go to see them, one afternoon. She had a somewhat cold reception from her mother, who has never shown any motherly feeling towards her. They never write to each other.

Mme. V. was put out to nurse at birth, as her mother did not like girls, and stayed there until she was three. She was in the same village as her mother, and used to see her and knew who she was, but the mother did nothing whatever for her, and paid no attention to her.

At three years of age her mother took her home, until she was twelve and a half, and this period was a very unhappy one for Mme. V. Her mother made her work very hard, was never satisfied, and practically ill-treated her. She used to beat her violently (the marks on her legs lasted for days), locked her up and did not always give her enough to eat, etc.

Mme. V. did not take her C.E.P. She 'had difficulty in learning', but stayed at school until she was twelve and a half. She was then placed on various farms until she was twenty. She remained a long time at one farm. The farmers were kind to her, helped her and were very fond of her. She still keeps in touch with them. She was working for them when, at a fête for returning prisoners of war, she met her husband, and they were attracted to each other. She was fond of him, but not deeply in love. They went about together; he used to come and see her on Sundays at her employers' house, and they advised her to marry him as he had a good reputation as a worker, like the rest of his family.

He once tried to have sexual relations with her, but she refused him, warning him that 'if it was only for "that" that he came to see her, he could be off!' He did not try again.

She went out for a time with another young man, whom she now regrets, as he is very steady and better than her husband.

Two days after the marriage, in December, 1945, M. V. revealed his true character, 'uncouth and coarse', telling his wife, for no reason at all, that she could go back home if she wished. Mme. V. cried about this, for she is very highly-strung, and laughs and cries with equal ease.

She is very active and animated, and has a loud, vivacious manner of talking. She is very vigorous in the way she runs her house. She always says just what she thinks—'it has to come out'—and she herself says she is a great talker. She must certainly have that reputation in the district.

However, Mme. V. has a kind heart and is very affectionate towards those who accept her affection, that is to say towards her children, and particularly the younger one, as the other is independent, is away from home all day and does not like being made a fuss of. She spoils the children, remembering her own unhappy childhood, and wishing to be a kind mother.

She is courageous and works hard. Her employers were always pleased with her, for she never stopped working even on Sundays. When she was pregnant with her first child, she hoed the beetroots almost up to the last day, until she could no longer keep on her feet. She is very active, needing to be occupied constantly. She does not sleep well; is restless, sleeps lightly and not for long. She has never been ill.

Mme. V. used to be a Public Assistance foster-mother. When Aimé was small, she looked after four foster-children at the same time, considering that it was no more difficult to look after five than one. She had a deep need of children. She is trying to get some more to look after at the moment. In spite of her possible love of children, it seems that Mme. V. may also be attracted by the idea of earning a little money in this way.

Mme. V. is of medium height, slim, with brown hair, clear bright eyes, and a rosy complexion. She seems to be of average intelligence; and is excessively emotional, with moods alternating between 'up' and 'down'. She cannot control herself and does not try to, being content to express thoughts and actions without restraint.

Her attitude towards her children is dominated by the memory of her unhappy childhood, and her mother's lack of affection. She dare not impose any discipline at all on her children for fear of frustrating them. She is a slave to them, and delights in it, making no attempt to modify her attitude, of which she is rather proud. She is possessive rather than dominating; but it seems that she will not be able to keep her children close to her for long. She is not upset by Aimé's detachment, perhaps because she still has Yves.

Having found no real satisfaction in her marriage, and later being deceived by her husband, she clings all the more to her children, and makes them the one interest in her life. She realizes that they will grow away from her very quickly, but she may herself not have the same feelings for them after they have reached a certain age.

Monsieur V.

Born 16th October, 1923, in a neighbouring village, of farming and land-owning parents, who now live in the same village as the son and his family.

His mother: aged 54; kind, but 'odd'. She may receive you well one day and rebuff you the next. Mme. V. gets on fairly well with her as she sees her only in the mornings, when she goes shopping.

His father: aged 55; in good health; a farmer. He is kind and affectionate; a heavy smoker.

231

They have had nine children, all living: eight boys and one girl. The eldest is M. V. with whom we are concerned.

His brothers:

(1) Aged 27; worked in a factory; has been ill for some months, with poisoning caused by working with coal.
(2) Aged 25; a farm-worker, healthy, but a heavy drinker.
(3) Aged 24; a road-worker; healthy; has been married for one year and lives in the same house as the V.s, in two adjoining rooms.
(4) Aged 22; a tractor-driver; good-natured.
(5) Aged 21; a farm-worker; is on military service.
(6) Aged 19; a farm-worker; healthy.
(7) Aged 15; a carter for his parents; 'pleasant—a good lad'.

A sister: Aged 18; lives with her parents, as she is considered 'very difficult' (even more so than the mother-in-law); she is spiteful and very contrary, but kind-hearted from time to time; we saw her and she was very pleasant and friendly, appearing to be quite intelligent.

None of them took the C.E.P. Apparently none of the family went to school very much, perhaps because they had to go to work early, perhaps because they lacked opportunity. The brothers and sister only get on moderately well together. They have no family feeling. Each lives his own life. Mme. V. does not seem to have a high opinion of her in-laws. She speaks of them with a certain amount of irony and contempt.

M. V. gets on well with his family. He started work at eleven years of age. He says he did well at school, but that he did not take his C.E.P. because he had to leave when he was eleven. At the moment he is a casual labourer, that is to say he is employed here or there on the farms according to the needs of the moment, hoeing beetroot, harvesting, wood-sawing, hay-making, etc. He seems to have spent a normal country childhood on his parents' farm. He has never been ill, apart from measles and chickenpox.

He is suspicious by nature—'no one knows what he is thinking'—does not talk much, is not affectionate but hard. He goes to work, returns for dinner, does not say a word, and goes out again. In the evening he plays a little with his children, but never has anything to say to his wife. They have no close ties with each other. He never goes out with her. He goes shooting, fishing, or to the cinema, or the neighbouring villages. This aroused his wife's suspicions several months ago. He used often to be absent, saying he was going to the cinema. Neighbours eventually took it upon themselves to tell Mme. V. of her husband's unfaithfulness. There were violent scenes, tears, threats of divorce, and now he seems to have settled down better; but the atmosphere is even more 'cold' than before. Mme. V. has stayed on because of the children, but she does not seem to have any further affection for her husband. She appears to have accepted her unsuccessful marriage.

M. V. has a tendency to drink, as have several of his brothers, but he has only been drunk occasionally in the last few months, before which there was a period when he drank heavily. He smokes also, one packet a day.

M. V. is of medium height and gives the impression of being robust; he is a country type, fair, slow-moving, slightly round-shouldered, unsmiling. He talks quite freely, but one feels that he is suspicious, though he unbends a little when speaking of his children, to whom he seems to be greatly attached.

There is no intimate relationship between M. and Mme. V. They are kept together solely by the children, whom they both love. M. V. did not want to have daughters; they are more difficult to bring up, and more costly; he is therefore very happy to have two 'lads'. He never punishes them; and is very gentle with them.

Mme. V. manages the budget; otherwise, she says, 'there would never be any money in the house'. She does not keep regular accounts; she considers that living is dear in the country, but she did not have much to say about this. One feels that it is not one of her daily problems. She will always 'manage to get by'. She has no spare-time interests, neither radio, nor reading nor entertainments. On Sundays, M. V. goes out shooting or on some other pursuit, and Mme. V. stays at home or visits her sister-in-law who lives in the same farmhouse. However, she is never bored. She is well adapted to life in the country, but wishes sometimes that there were more amusements.

Aimé

Born at full term, 9th July, 1947, at home.

No difficulties during pregnancy, which was welcomed; the parents hoped for a boy; occasional vomiting up to six months.

Weight at birth: 4·500 kg. (9 lb. 14 oz.); a normal confinement; immediate cry.

Breast-fed solely up to thirteen months; first thickened feeds given at thirteen months in a spoon. He was very hungry at that time, and there was no difficulty in weaning him.

First tooth: at four months (six teeth at six months).

Words: at six months. ⎫
Sentences: at one year? ⎬ was very precocious.
Walked: at ten months. ⎭

233

He is very well developed. Mme. V. has had no difficulty about his food, nor about his sleep (he has always slept well), nor even about his cleanliness.

She put him on the pot at eight months and he very quickly started to ask to do his duty in the pot. He appears to have been clean by day and by night at one year.

He was a nice baby, and good-natured when small, but since the birth of his brother he is 'not easy'. He is very jealous.

He did not seem to be much affected at the time of the birth. His mother told him that she was going to buy a little sister in the town. Her stay at the maternity hospital was explained by a broken leg. When she came back he asked to see this broken leg, but he was told that it was better and that there was now nothing to see.

Mme. V. thinks that he is too small to understand, and that in any case she would never have dared to tell him anything on this subject. She seems embarrrassed. When he shows jealousy, she either does not answer, or tells him that she loves each of them as much as the other.

He is inclined to sulk and she lets him do so. She does not punish him, but just shouts, threatens him, raises her hand, but does not strike him. When she has had too much, she cries.

Aimé is 'disagreeable', she says; he takes after his father. One day when she was tired, she told him she would go away and leave him; he replied 'That's all right; I'll stay with papa, who will get another wife'. This reply hurt Mme. V. very much, and she cried for a long time; there were tears in her eyes as she was telling about it.

He does not go to school yet, but disappears all day long. As a rule, he has lunch with his grandmother, without telling his mother beforehand. He returns home late in the evening. His mother lets him do as he likes. She does not try to keep him with her; she could not do so. She feels that she is a slave to this child, as she is to the other one also, for that matter.

Aimé is very attractive, slight, fair, with blue eyes and very active. He runs about everywhere, preferably in the dirt. He goes into the fields with his paternal uncles, and seems to be very fond of them and of his grandparents, with whom he practically lives, since he only goes home for his dinner and to sleep, when he does not actually sleep at his grandparents' house.

Yves

Born after full-term pregnancy at the Montereau Maternity Hospital, 19th November, 1950. Normal pregnancy, wanted, no trouble; the mother worked right up to the last moment.

She had not considered the possibility of having a boy—it was to be a girl; hence there was inevitable disappointment, followed by acceptance.

Forceps delivery, the child had a misshapen skull for some days. Mme. V. suffered a great deal; she had a thrombosis after returning home. She was not well for several months after the confinement.

Immediate cry; weight: 4·250 kg. (9 lb. 6 oz.).

Breast-fed up to seven and a half months. Mme. V. would have liked to feed him longer, like the first child, but she had no more milk. She thinks that she has not properly recovered from her confinement; is still tired.

She gave six feeds regularly, every three hours; no feeds at night as the baby slept well.

First thickened feed, in a bottle, at seven and a half months. Took it well, no difficulties.

First solids at ten months; he has fed himself at the table since he was one year old.

First smile: at two months.

First tooth: at eight months.

Could sit up at five–six months.

Walked: at ten months.

Feeding: Mme. V. has never had any trouble with Yves, as he has always eaten anything. He has a good appetite, and when he wants something he is given it even between his normal meal-times. Up to the time he was weaned, she kept to a fairly strict time-table, but since then it is he who has the say. He is always hungry, and 'would go and eat the animals' food if he was not prevented from doing so'.

At the present, he has:

In the morning: a patent food, bread and butter.

At midday: the same as his parents, vegetables, meat, fruit. He eats a whole beefsteak.

At 2 p.m.: before his sleep, a bottle of milk.

At 4 p.m.: a slice of bread and butter and a bottle of milk.

At 6 p.m.: soup and an egg; and another bottle when he goes to bed at 9 p.m.

Sleep: Has always had deep, tranquil sleep. Mme. V. rocks him for five minutes sometimes before putting him to bed, and to start with he sleeps in his parents' bed with them. When he is sound asleep, she puts him in his own bed. It is he who has established this practice.

He does not suck anything, neither thumb nor dummy, which seems to displease his mother.

Cleanliness: He was put on the pot from ten months, and used to be left there for a quarter of an hour or twenty minutes, but he would do nothing until afterwards. Now he asks to go on the pot. He stays there sometimes for an hour, playing, urinates and eventually has a motion, but more often he does it afterwards in his knickers. In the evening he is put on the pot after dinner, and then he performs regularly.

For micturition: he either wets his knickers during the day or asks for his pot. But at night, for the last two or three months, he has hardly ever wet the bed. His father takes him up in the morning.

Whatever happens, the mother never says anything, as she thinks he is too young. She never shows him his urine or his stools, which he deposits anywhere. He did it twice during one of our visits; she simply washes him.

Play: Yves is full of play, will amuse himself with anything, has no toys apart from a large teddy-bear, which he takes to bed, and a rubber ball. He plays by himself or with his brother.

He is a lovely fair child, chubby and rosy, smiling, friendly and uninhibited. He played with coins, and clung to his mother, who likes to carry him, fondling him and kissing him.

He plays 'the spoilt child'. When he wants something he has a little fit of temper if his mother does not give in to him straight away, then he gets it. He often gets into a temper, and rolls on the floor: she lets him do it or gives him a gentle slap. He is very affectionate towards his parents and his brother.

Yves spends a lot of time with his grandparents, like his brother, for in the afternoons Mme. V. often works with her husband. At present she is cutting and stacking wood. She was doing that when we had our last interview with her. Her husband and her sister-in-law, who had shown us the way, were both there also.

Mme. V. wondered why we were coming to see her again, and what else she could tell us. She had been very frank the first time, but one must not ask too much of her. She had had enough; however, she received us cordially.

When Mme. V. is working out-of-doors, Yves goes to his grandparents and his aunt of eighteen looks after him. She is very fond of him, but does not let him do as he pleases like his mother, and he is more obedient with her. All the family seem to think that Mme. V. is too weak with her children and that she lets them do anything they like. Another sister-in-law whom we saw was also of this opinion, and makes a point of being strict with Yves when his mother is not there.

Yves is very fond of his brother; he often goes to him, but Aimé does not always welcome him. He is very often out-of-doors, in all weathers, even when it is very cold; Mme. V. puts plenty of clothes on him and he plays in the yard.

Both children are in excellent physical health, and seem at present to have benefited from the warm affectionate atmosphere, and freedom from constraint, in which they have been brought up. They are bright, natural, friendly and very active.

However, the family equilibrium seems somewhat precarious, between Mme V., whose conduct is motivated by her experiences in childhood, and M. V., whose role in the family life is limited to being present and showing affection to the children. There appears to be no positive force linking the parents, and the children will doubtless react to this lack of unity by exploiting it.

Aimé is already capricious, uncooperative, a family tyrant, and his little brother Yves is progressively becoming the same. However, the life in the country, and the nearness of the grandparents and their family, lessen the difficulties, as the children are able to pass their time in two different atmospheres.

EXAMINATION OF DEVELOPMENT

Dr. Marcelle Geber

Yves V.   Born on 19th *October,* 1950
Examined February, 1952 (15 *months old*).

The examination was carried out in a large country kitchen.

This room is on a level with the yard, in which Yves was playing when we arrived.

The interior is well kept.

When we arrived, Mme. V. was preparing the midday meal (11 a.m.) and her sister-in-law (husband's sister) was sewing.

Mme. V. received us rather coolly at first, saying that it was very late, that her husband would soon be home, and that he would not want to have to wait for his lunch. 'As far as he's concerned, things have to be on time, he likes to eat at exactly the right time, and everything has to be just so.'

When we suggested coming back after the meal, she relented, insisted on our going in, and went to fetch Yves.

After this, Mme. V. replied directly and quite graciously to the questions we asked about Yves' development. She also told us that she adored children, and had looked after five from the Public Assistance before he was born. She wanted to have some more to look after.

Mme. V. is a young woman who speaks volubly, becomes animated, and gets flushed; she was somewhat embarrassed at the beginning, then little by little became more at ease. She seems to fear her husband's authoritative attitude.

Appearance

Yves is a fair little boy, chubby, with an animated face and a wide-awake expression. His skin is clear, rosy, his mucous membranes in good condition, his hair silky.

He is in excellent health. He gives the impression of being strong. He looks at a stranger with a lively interest and is immediately at ease, chattering and saying a few words.

TEST

Seated on a chair at the table, he took an immediate interest in the test objects. He was particularly interested in the cubes, which he put in and out of the cup. He refused to let them be taken away from him. When he was offered another object he said '*non-non*' and shook his head. It was only after he had been allowed to play for about ten minutes with the cubes, putting them into the cup, taking them out again, holding them out to me but immediately taking them back again, that he gradually became interested in the bottle and the lozenge. He put it into the bottle very quickly, got it out, and laughed. After that he readily accepted the succession of tests.

His interest was keen, and he took great pleasure in the test. He was very animated, laughing, and turning towards the examiner, his mother and his aunt.

He was absorbed for a long time in the book, stroking the pictures, choosing the ones he liked, naming some of the animals.

He protested when the test was finished, but was then quite happy with the doctor, who immediately took over.

(1) Development

His development is, on the whole, in advance of that of a child of his age, especially in locomotion and social reactions.

(a) Motor

> Locomotion: He walks, and runs quickly but still unsteadily, squats on his heels to play, kicks a rubber ball, seats himself in the little chair, climbs on a large chair, climbs and descends stairs when he is held by one hand. His muscles feel well-developed, firm, good tone, and he walks, runs and plays with noticeable strength. His mother told us that he has walked

238

since he was one year old, and that he is always playing and running about. His motor development is very advanced, and corresponds to that of a child of nineteen and a half months. L.Q. = 128.

Manual dexterity: Yves is left-handed. Mme. V. told us that several members of her family were left-handed. She leaves him free to use whichever hand he pleases.

He shows no abnormalities of prehension. He grasped the cubes very well, took the lozenge between the thumb and index finger, helped to turn the pages, threw the ball. His development is that of a child of sixteen and a half months. M.Q. = 109.

(b) Adaptivity

He made a tower of three or four bricks easily and quickly, put the ten cubes into the cup and took them out again, placed the lozenge in the bottle and immediately got it out again by turning the bottle upside down. He made a tower of three blocks. He scribbled spontaneously, with great delight, and copied a line. All these actions were performed quickly, and with precision, and here again his development is on the whole superior to that of a child of his age: eighteen months. A.Q. = 118.

(c) Language

It is in this sphere that Yves is the least advanced.

Expression: He can say a dozen words, including the names of persons, but does not really talk baby-talk; he seems to begin with baby-talk but end with words pronounced clearly. His verbal expression is that of a child of fifteen and a half months. E.Q. = 102.

Comprehension: He fondles the pictures, looks at them and chooses those he likes best. His mother told us that he loves books. His level here is that of sixteen months. C.Q. = 105.

(d) Personal-Social

He can feed himself, gets himself dirty, turns his utensils upside down. He holds out his empty plate. He holds his cup well. He has as yet no control of his sphincters.

He pulls an adult along to show him something. He likes dragging a toy behind him and carrying a doll.

239

He is therefore, on the whole, advanced in self-feeding and play, but retarded in sphincter control. His mother has put him on the pot since he was ten months, and has smacked him when he made a mess on the floor indoors, but does not say anything when he does it out-of-doors.

With regard to feeding and play, his reactions correspond to a level of maturation of twenty months, and of fifty-six weeks for his sphincter, which represents a level of eighteen and a half months as far as his personal-social maturity is concerned. P.S.Q. = 121.

(2) *Behaviour*

(*a*) *When faced with a new situation:*

Yves accepted our visit very well, and was immediately at ease. He came and sat himself down at the table when he was shown the cubes.

(*b*) *Towards objects:*

His interest was spontaneous and very lively. He participated very actively in the test, handling the objects with pleasure, laughing, talking gibberish, with a few distinct words.

However, he refused to accept the succession of objects and had to be allowed to keep the cubes for about ten minutes. It is true that, owing to the mother's attitude on our arrival, the test was begun very quickly, before establishing rapport and gaining the child's confidence. These ten minutes of play with the cubes correspond, therefore, to the procedure necessary to fulfil the conditions of the test, in which the adult has to demand certain things from the child, which he can obtain only if he has managed to gain the child's confidence sufficiently.

After this play, which the examiner permitted, the child accepted the other objects, and showed just as much interest and pleasure in them as in the cubes.

(*c*) *Towards strange adults:*

He accepted the strangers immediately, smiled at us, and was at his ease. He looked at the examiner with pleasure and satisfaction when shown the first objects, which were the cubes. But he resisted when, having performed the required actions, the examiner wished to take the cubes away from him. However, the examiner being permissive of the child's play, he made use of her a great deal, holding out the objects to her, talking to her, smiling, laughing, attracting her attention.

(*d*) *Towards his parents:*

He made use of his mother and his aunt, calling them, laughing, showing them what he had done.

(3) *The Mother*

and aunt participated in the child's activities, watched him, answered his smiles, encouraged him to do even better.

Conclusion

This child's development is clearly superior to that of his chronological age: D.Q. = 114. This is explained by the favourable conditions in which he lives. He has room to play, is out-of-doors most of the time. His parents love their children; they are interested in the child, play with him, encourage him to talk, show him pictures, allow him plenty of freedom.

His behaviour is also satisfactory. He trusts adults, from whom he expects only pleasant things, and he is quite happy to let an adult direct his actions, if he is considerate.

PHYSICAL EXAMINATION

Dr. Cyrille Koupernik

Yves V. Born 19th October, 1950
Examined 23rd February, 1952 (at the age of 16 months).

Previous History

The mother's second confinement.
Her elder son is four years old.
She has never had a miscarriage.

Pregnancy: Mme. V. did not vomit during her pregnancy; fewer foetal movements than during the first pregnancy.

Confinement: At the maternity hospital in the neighbouring town. Full-term pregnancy, birth weight 4.250 gm. (9 lb. 6 oz.); labour lasted eight hours. The mother was given chloroform; forceps delivery. She does not know whether the child was cyanozed or jaundiced at birth, or if he cried immediately.

First days: During the first days he had severe icterus. He had no difficulty with sucking; he was neither specially sleepy nor, on the other hand, restless.

It should be noticed that the mother had a pulmonary embolus on the third day of the puerperium.

First development:
First smile at a human face: at three months.
Voluntary prehension: early (no more precise information).
Head movement: early.

241

Sitting up: early.

Walked at ten months.

Toilet-training: is not yet clean during the day; is put on the pot, waits to be lifted off, and then does it alongside. When he wants to urinate puts his hand to his knickers. On the other hand, he is dry most nights. Toilet-training was started at the age of nine months.

First word: 'papa', at eight months. Began to understand words towards the age of one year.

First tooth at eight months (now has nine teeth).

The child was put in the care of his aunt and grandmother during the first month, because of the mother's illness. The aunt still continues to help with him.

No history of previous illness; no convulsions or screaming attacks.

Vaccinated against smallpox, successfully, and without any specific reaction, at the age of seven months.

His mother is twenty-seven years old, healthy, normal menstruation; nothing of note in her personal or family history.

The father is twenty-eight years old, equally healthy; nothing of note in his personal or family history.

A brother, four years old, healthy, normal development.

Present State

Yves walks without difficulty, and runs.

He prefers to use his left hand; as do his brother and a paternal uncle.

Play: He plays with his teddy-bear, which he calls Tintin; makes him dance, takes him to bed.

He plays equally happily with a little barrow that he wheels along. He likes to tear paper and pretends to read the newspaper.

He still has a tendency to throw and break things.

Comprehension and language: He understands, according to his mother, most of the ordinary words, all simple orders, knows what everyday things are for.

He often takes people by the hand to show them things or to get them to give him something.

He chatters constantly, and says about a dozen words. He dances to the radio. He enjoys making funny faces at himself in the mirror.

Habits: He sleeps in his parents' room.

He is not frightened of the dark, of animals, doctors, fire, space, or water. He is a little frightened of motor-cars.

He has no trouble over food; prefers sweet things.

He gets into a temper, rolls on the ground but never goes in for breath-holding.

He is not shy with strangers.

He is equally affectionate with mother and father; shows no preference for men or for women. He loves children.

He does not suck his thumb, nor rock himself.

Physical Examination

The mother does not know his present weight. He does not see a doctor regularly. He is a bonny, fair child with rosy cheeks, and hazel eyes. His head circumference is 51 cm., with no sign of deformity, and there are no signs of rickets.

When standing, he has an excellent posture with firm muscles, but, when lifted from a lying position to a sitting position, he has a slight relaxation of the muscles of the right side of the abdomen.

No hernia, nor ectopic testicle.

He has a certain degree of normal hypotonus.

The tendon reflexes are normal and the plantar-skin reflex is bilaterally flexor.

5. THE M. FAMILY
(*Farmers*)
Mme. Laurette Amado

The M. family consists of the mother, 28½ years old; the father, 36½; and their two daughters, Chantal, nearly 6, and Marie-Claude, 21 months.

They farm a large holding outside the village, yielding a portion of the produce to the owner instead of paying rent.

A number of large buildings make up 'the farm'. The house has six rooms. We only saw the very large, well-kept kitchen, which contains a large table, four benches, chairs, a white stove, a box for wood, an immense frigidaire hidden by cretonne curtains, a wireless set and a sink with running water. There is electricity (power), but no gas.

They have a dining-room and four bedrooms, one for the parents, one for the girls, and the others, no doubt, for the staff.

They have a maid, who does not sleep on the farm, and farm hands, three or four in winter and about ten in summer.

They all have meals together in the kitchen. Mme. M. prepares the meals, and all eat the same food, as M. M. does not like to have any dishes different from those given to his employees. Mme. M. thinks they might do so occasionally, but her husband refuses. Only the children have specially cooked food, though eating at table with the others.

It is a large farm, of more than 100 hectares, though Mme. M. gives us no details about this, nor about the stock. They sell milk, butter and eggs to the villagers.

They own a four-seater Vivaquatre Renault car.

Madame M.

Born on the 6th June, 1923, in a neighbouring village.

Her father: 79 years old, formerly a baker; has had very good health; does not drink; very pleasant.

Her mother: 66 years old, also formerly a baker; she was a widow of the 1914 war, and had three sons when she married Mme. M.'s father.

The old people live in a village not far from Mme. M., who sees them regularly, and often writes.

Mme. M.'s three half-brothers are older than she, and left home early, so that she was brought up as an only child. She is on good terms with her brothers, who have 'good jobs' in Paris, and they write to each other. All three are married and have children.

Mme. M.'s mother is pleasant, affectionate, a very good mother. She is very meticulous. She is a cardiac subject, with hypertension, has been under medical care for two years and has consulted a well-known specialist in Paris. Mme. M. is unceasingly worried about her.

It was a contented household, there were no quarrels, and Mme. M. had a happy childhood.

At first she lived with her parents, then, when she was about twelve, she was sent to a convent school as a boarder, her parents being devout Catholics. She has happy memories of her four years of boarding school. The Sisters were kind, and Mme. M. bore their discipline very well. She thinks it a necessary part of a good education.

She worked well, only having a certain amount of difficulty with arithmetic and algebra. At about sixteen she gained a certificate of secondary studies, which, however, is not official. She also passed obligatory sporting tests, but did not care very much for sport. She was a 'good girl' who gave no trouble to her parents or teachers, and she had many friends.

She first menstruated at thirteen. Her mother had never prepared her for this and she was told about it by school-friends.

After boarding school, Mme. M. studied shorthand-typing and bookkeeping. Her parents wanted her to have a career and she agreed. She found it hard to learn, but wanted to succeed, and worked hard. She was living with her parents then, and took courses at Sens three times a week. She often went to Paris to visit her brothers during this period. Her parents allowed her a great deal of freedom, as they trusted her. Nevertheless, they would never have allowed her to go to a dance alone and 'come home at four in the morning, as young girls do nowadays'.

She never worked as a shorthand-typist because the war came, and her parents preferred to keep her at home because of the air raids and food shortages, which did not affect them in the country. She therefore stayed at home until, at a wedding, she met her future husband.

They went about together for a time, and were married in April, 1946. They then came to live on the farm where they are now, which was then managed by M. M.'s father. Mme. M. took well to her new life, as she loves quiet and the country, and is never bored. She has no time to be. She looks after her little girls, the cooking, often the chickens, ducks, etc., and in the summer, the garden. She also looks after everything to do with the social insurance of the staff. If a Sunday comes when she can be alone she enjoys it very much, because the rest of the time she is among so many people which, she says, is tiring.

She needs plenty of activity. The house is remarkably well kept and she and her daughters very clean; she is clearly scrupulous in every way.

She is rather cold and stiff in appearance, not smiling easily, not saying more than she can help, and no doubt not wanting to give too much away about herself, her household, the farm, etc. She is of medium height, thin, with dark hair beginning to go grey. She looked very smart in a very clean, bright, coloured overall. She is quite attractive, but too much on the defensive, and unwilling to unbend. Very emotional and blushes easily.

At the first meeting she was very much annoyed at our intrusion into her affairs, but later agreed to our work on our promising that there would be nothing to sign, that there would be no inquiry about the social insurance, and that she would not be forced to show her children to the Public Health doctor who comes with a van once a month, and whom she never consults as she considers the children to be in good health.

On our first visit we were not able to be alone with her, her parents-in-law and a friend having arrived at almost the same time as ourselves. The visit was therefore passed in an atmosphere of coming and going of men, and in the presence of the mother-in-law, who took an active part in the conversation.

At the second visit, Mme. M. was more friendly, but she did not send away the maid, who sat doing the mending alongside us, though without entering into the conversation. Only at the end, when it was time to shut the hens up or fetch the milk, were we able to have a few minutes alone with Mme. M., though she did not becc me any more confiding.

We are of the opinion that more frequent meetings would not have produced more information and certainly not more confidences. Mme. M. seems to be mistrustful by nature, and does not allow herself to soften easily. We felt that she was all the time on the defensive.

Mistrustful to the end, she refused to allow the doctor to come and examine her daughter physically and psychologically. She was most definite about this, and worried at the thought of anyone coming near her daughter. We did not insist.

Monsieur M.

Born the 24th August, 1915, in a neighbouring village, the only son of farmers.

His father: 64 years old, in good health.

A farmer, he rented and worked large farms, like the one where his son now is, and which he himself ran till a few years ago. He now lives in a house he has bought, four kilometres from his son. He is very pleasant and distinguished-looking, not of the usual peasant type. He makes one feel that he is well off, and that he has contacts in towns. His clothes are well looked after; he wore a very clean fur-lined jacket. He has a car, which allows him to visit his children frequently.

His mother: 57 years old, in good health.

A very pleasant woman. She has only the one son, to whom she is very much attached.

She is tall, with a fine, distinguished face; and during our first meeting she talked a lot, and approvingly, about her little grand-daughters.

M. M. takes after his mother very much. He is tall and slight, with fine regular features. He is very distinguished, very quiet, gentle, but rather cold, perhaps from shyness. It was not possible to have any private conversation with him, but in any case, a contact established for a few minutes would have produced insignificant results. He seems to talk very little.

He is 'easy', Mme. M. says, easily pleased, never reproachful, never raises his voice. One feels he is a strong man, honest, good, just, but also reserved, living very much within himself.

He seems to have had an easy childhood, the only child of parents with a happy home. He gained his C.E.P. Worked well in school, but wanted to farm with his father rather than stay on there.

At the outbreak of war, he was finishing his military service; was a prisoner in Germany for five years, and was therefore away from his family for seven years altogether, except for one six-months' leave before the war. In Germany he was not very unhappy, at least physically, for he worked on a farm, and he quickly re-adjusted on his return.

Soon after this, he met his future wife at a wedding. After a serious courtship of six months, they were married in April, 1946, and settled down on the farm with M. M.'s parents. The latter retired shortly afterwards, leaving the working of the farm to their son. It is certainly a happy home, but there seems to be little intimacy. The couple seem rather independent of each other, each having a separate part to play. M. M. manages the farm, which entails hard work as he has high standards and wants the farm to pay. Mme. M. busies herself with the house, the staff and the children. The one has to be out-doors all the time, the other in the house.

They never have meals by themselves, but always with the maid and the farm-hands. On Sunday, he goes shooting and in the winter they go, by car, to visit the parents of the one or the other. In summer there is even more work, and never any holidays. Mme. M. is rarely

247

alone, but puts up with this well. They went to Paris for two days in February (their last trip was in 1947), but did not take the car as garages in Paris are too expensive. The noise and bustle tired them and they were pleased to return to the country. They were struck by the 'debauchery' they saw in a café: young girls with old men or vice-versa, no married couples, it seemed, only couples having a casual affair.

The budget is in the hands of Mme. M., who is probably very economical. They are certainly rich, but hide the fact carefully, and the restraint we noticed was no doubt due to fear of having to broach questions of money, which we had to avoid.

Chantal

Born at full term, 4th June, 1947, at home. Mme. M.'s mother came to look after her daughter.

Easy pregnancy; a wanted child; no fatigue; no vomiting.

Normal birth, but umbilical cord looped around the neck; immediate cry.

Weight: 3·500 kg.

Breast-fed for three months; seven feeds, one at night; a breast abscess; one bottle given at fifteen days so as not to tire Mme. M. Feeding schedules adhered to very strictly, within a minute.

Chantal cried all night for three months, from evening till morning; nothing would calm her. They tried everything: leaving her alone, soothing, rocking, giving her a drink. The doctor remarked that she turned night into day. During the day she was good-tempered.

When one night, suddenly, she stopped this crying, Mme. M. realized, afterwards, that Chantal had sucked her thumb from that moment.

Smiled: at two months.

First tooth: at twelve months.

First words: at eight–nine months.

First sentences: at one and a half years.

Walked: at one year.

Appetite: small, nothing tempted her. Mme. M. did not force her as she appeared to be developing normally and looked extremely well. She therefore did not insist on her eating more than she wanted. At eighteen months she ate alone, with a spoon.

She drinks a lot of milk, and at four years would still like a bottle. Her mother broke her of this abruptly.

Cleanliness attained at two years—put on the pot from one year.

Has never been ill, except for slight colds.

Sleep regular but rather light, from 8.30 at night to 7.30 in the morning.

Has always sucked her thumb, but is made to feel ashamed of it; does not suck it in public.

Plays with her dolls, her ball, but above all at dressing up; is very vain. Likes playing with her sister.

Not easily made angry, very gentle, sweet, affectionate, very sensitive, cries easily, gets upset, blushes. She is a little jealous of her small sister. At the time of her sister's birth she was with her paternal grandparents. She asked no questions, and was told nothing about it. 'She is too little', and in any case Mme. M. would have been very embarrassed. She thinks these things are learned outside, little by little, and does not plan to give her daughters any sexual education. She thinks, too, that on the farm they will have plenty of opportunity of learning the truth from animals. Chantal often speaks of the cock mounting the hen, but they pay no attention.

Mme. M. has no difficulty with her daughter, who is very pretty, slight, with a high colour, very bright blue eyes. She is smiling and placid, and played alone very quietly during our visit. Not demanding and not shy, except when her mother talked to us about her.

She sleeps alone since her sister's birth, but is rather timid.

She goes to a nursery school, four kilometres away, in the village where her paternal grandparents live; she stays with them and they take her back to her parents on Wednesday and Saturday nights. The school in their own village does not take children under six, and Mme. M. wanted to put her to school earlier.

She has settled down well at school, it seems; is very happy to go, and 'works' well. She very much likes staying with her grandparents, but is a bit upset on leaving home and delighted to return. She does not like leaving her little sister, of whom she is jealous, with her mother.

Marie-Claude

Full term child, born 19th May, 1950.

Normal pregnancy, wanted, no sickness or fatigue.

Birth at home, normal, but umbilical cord looped as with Chantal; immediate cry.

Weight: 4·250 kg.

Breast-fed till nine months. Five breast-feeds, supplemented by one bottle in the afternoon to give Mme. M. freedom. Five breast-feeds and a bottle at night up to one year. She cried at night, though less than her sister, and the bottle quietened her. She weaned herself.

First smile: at two months.

First tooth: at thirteen months. She has twelve now.

Walked: at fifteen months.

First words: at eight months. Uses baby-talk but now begins to form sentences, understands everything, makes herself understood.

Wore swaddling-clothes during the day for the first month, and still wears them at night because of the cold.

Feeding: never had any difficulties, always hungry, eats everything. At present has four meals a day:

Morning: milk, bread and butter.

Noon: at table, has fed herself since the age of eighteen months; vegetables, meat, fruit.

Four o'clock: a glass of milk, a slice of bread and butter.

Evening: soup, sweet.

Very exact schedules, especially when she was little. She waits without crying.

Cleanliness: was put on the pot from when she was between one year and thirteen months old. Very quickly learnt to use it and has been clean for two–three months. She asks for the pot for bowel evacuation as well as to urinate.

She still wets her bed at night, which her mother thinks normal; and she is waiting, without scolding, for her to grow out of it.

Sleep: peaceful and regular, from 8.30 at night to 7.30 in the morning. Also in the afternoons, from 2–4 precisely. If she is still sleeping at that time, she is awakened; and if she is awake she is left in bed till 4, when, invariably, Mme. M. goes to get her up. She does not suck her thumb, has never been rocked, has never been ill.

Play: she plays alone or with her sister. Plays with her doll or with anything; imitates her sister a lot, and is beginning to dress up with her.

Mme. M. has no difficulties with Marie-Claude. She has an easier nature than her sister, is 'less nervous', does not get into tempers, does not cry; on the contrary, she is always laughing, good humoured, and complacent.

She is a pretty little brunette with big dark eyes and a high colour, who smiles very freely, and behaved very well during our visits. She is plump, seems to be in excellent health.

Mme. M. is very satisfied with her two daughters, whom she loves equally.

Up till now she has had to do very little punishing (one smack to Chantal only), and yet, she says, her daughters obey her. She never gives in unless they cry. Mme. M. cannot bear to hear them cry, and thinks they are too young to be allowed to cry. She therefore gives them what they want when they come to the point of tears, which seems to be fairly seldom.

Mme. M. wants her daughters to be well brought up. She will give them a religious education such as she received herself. She has not yet thought about what her girls might do later.

She has no difficulties in her maternal role. Her daughters have brought themselves up 'by themselves' since birth, and she thinks this is likely to continue. She knows, however, that it may not always be easy.

She is very strict, but on account of her many duties, her children enjoy a certain freedom.

Her husband takes no part in the upbringing of his children, leaving this entirely to his wife. He plays with his daughters, and is very gentle with them.

To sum up, the M. family seems to us very well integrated, and well adapted to their social status. The mother is fairly rigid, but the father's gentleness, and life in the country in good conditions, allows the children to develop well.

NOTE: Owing to the mother's unwillingness, it was not possible for the children to do the Gesell Test, or to be examined by the doctor.

Part Three

BRITISH

CASE

HISTORIES

THE BRITISH CASE HISTORIES

Louise Mestel

The cases from the United Kingdom were by no means intended to present a clear and detailed account of a well-established research programme, but were the results of the first six months' work on a project of study of the training of babies in Leeds. The field is enormous and important: no one has yet studied how Leeds mothers actually handle their babies, and the advice of local experts on baby care shows, to say the least, considerable variety.

The project was based on a questionnaire, drafted by a Committee drawn from interested university departments. This draft was used in two ways. First, it was circulated to a small group of university mothers, chosen for their willing co-operation and their interest in the problem, who gave their answers in writing. It was clear that these results would have no statistical significance, but certain interesting features of the replies were mentioned by Professor MacCalman in a lecture at the Seminar. (See Vol. I, p. 71).

Secondly, the questionnaire was used orally with the mothers of selected children. Two cases were chosen from the records of the Child Guidance Clinic, and the questions put to these mothers by a psychiatric social worker and a psychologist. For purposes of comparison, two mothers of 'normal' children were also interviewed; the children had been matched with the 'abnormal' for age, intelligence, family structure, locality, ethnic group, and social and income levels. In all cases, a brief description of the parents' background has been given, and, in the 'abnormal' cases, the clinic's records were summarized. As it happened, one 'normal' child appeared to be well-adjusted, while the other showed signs of disturbance.

The questionnaire was not used exactly in its written form. Explanations of ambiguous points had to be made, tactful re-phrasings were often necessary, and some sections, dealing with subjects taboo in the normal conversation of strangers, were given only after the barriers had been gently broken down with such topics as Speech, Health or Games. However, very great care was taken to keep the conversation emotionally neutral: the questioner's asides were intended only to make the atmosphere more friendly and relaxed, and not to twist a meaning or suggest that one answer would meet with greater approval than another.

The answers were taken down, as far as possible, as the mother spoke them, and her own turns of phrase retained. They were presented for discussion in the form of a continuous autobiography; this was purely a literary device, to avoid the repetition of the questionnaire (or a constant need for the reader at the Seminar to refer to it separately), and also to try to lend a touch of life and humanity. In no case has anything been changed, inserted or left out.

Now that the committee's questionnaire has been tried out in practice, it is possible to see that several changes would be needed in any future work. Throughout, however, there was no thought of planning a rigorous survey, or even of making an exhaustive study of one or two cases.

The two British children, whose cases are presented in detail in this volume, were studied and recorded according to the normal child guidance practice of multi-disciplinary examination by psychiatrist, psychologist and psychiatric social worker, operating as a team.

1. PETER

(This account by Peter's mother, Mrs. R., was compiled from her answers to the Leeds Questionnaire)

UPBRINGING FOR THE FIRST TWO YEARS

(1) *Mother's Attitude towards having Children*

I first found out that I could have children at the age of eleven. I felt very bewildered at the knowledge, but my feelings have naturally changed since then.

I was very surprised when I found I was pregnant, as we had been married fifteen years without having a child, although we had tried deliberately to have one ever since we married. My first feelings were very happy feelings towards having a baby, and I looked forward very much to being a mother. My husband and my family were very pleased too.

The idea of never having children would certainly have worried me. I think eventually we should have adopted one.

If health and income allowed, I would like to have two children.

I can't think of any drawbacks about having children.

There weren't exactly any medical difficulties about having children in my case, except that I did not conceive as quickly as I had hoped.

(2) *Mother's Experiences during Pregnancy*

I felt exceptionally well during pregnancy, and only had very slight morning sickness during the second month. I knew how the child would be born, and looked on it just as a natural experience. I was neither proud nor embarrassed by my size.

The child showed a lot of activity in the later months of pregnancy.

Being a housewife, there was little change in my usual routine. There was little change in diet; after about four months I couldn't wear most of my clothes and had to wear loose garments. There was no intercourse during most of the pregnancy. I felt that good food, fresh air and resting when I was tired, would be good for the baby; shocks of any sort would be bad. My husband didn't exactly have to make any changes in behaviour because of my pregnancy; but he was more considerate to me and helped with my household duties, etc.

No instruction was given me about the development of the child or the stages of labour, but I was given some instruction about looking after the baby. I read the book *Parentcraft* (published by the National

Association for Maternal and Child Welfare), which I found very helpful.

(3) *Birth*

All of us looked on labour pains as natural and inevitable. Anaesthetics were used, and I was unconscious when my baby arrived. The birth took place at a nursing home, with a lady gynaecologist in attendance. There was no one else I would have liked to be present. In my case, I would describe childbirth as a painful experience. I had to have an episiotomy and also had a lateral *placenta praevia*, and as a result I was ill.

Peter was separated from me at birth.

More expenditure was required at this time, because of the nursing-home and specialist's fees, and also the expense of the things required for the baby.

There was no death in the family round about this time.

Peter was quite normal at birth, except for a bruised forehead caused by the use of instruments. These bruises soon faded away. My recovery was rather protracted, owing to such a bad confinement.

Peter wasn't christened, as we are Jews, but he was circumcised.

(4) *Feeding*

I remember it was more than half a day after his birth when I first fed Peter. He was breast-fed, of course; I think it's healthier and you avoid messing about with bottles. I must say it was a wonderful experience for me, and when I had finished feeding him and put him down to sleep, my arms felt quite empty. I should say he fed normally; he wasn't either greedy or slow. I held him in my arms, in the usual way.

I started off feeding him at fixed intervals, on the advice of the nurses in the nursing home. Later I found I could relax it a little.

He never refused food. I usually saw that he spent about twenty minutes over each feed.

I started including orange and black-currant juice in his feeds at about two months. He wouldn't take them from a bottle at all, so I tried a cup and spoon right from the start. It wasn't a success at all to begin with, but by four months he could put the cup to his lips without making too much mess.

I had to wean him very suddenly, at a moment's notice, as I developed septic tonsillitis when he was six months old. He was cutting his first tooth at about that time. The amount of milk had decreased beforehand, and he didn't seem to miss the breast at all.

When he was teething, I gave him rusks, but he couldn't hold them and kept dropping them. He had a teething-ring instead. He never had a dummy. He started sucking his thumb when he was about nine months old and it went on till he began to walk at eighteen months. I didn't like to see it, but on the doctor's advice I tried to realize it was a comfort to him. I didn't do anything to stop it—just pulled his thumb out of his mouth when he fell asleep.

Solids were first introduced at four and a half months. I fed them to him by spoon.

He was usually fed by himself, but his father used to be around at the time. He often attended meals with my mother, especially Saturday lunches. Saturday lunch is quite a special occasion in Jewish families.

Meal-times were regular, and he didn't have much in between meals—perhaps a drink, that's all. I can't say we had any trouble over food; he was a good eater until he was two. The difficulties came later! He never over-ate, either.

I thought cream-buns and fancy cakes were bad for him; if he had anything like that it was plain and home-made. I didn't give him sweets at that age. Good foods, I thought, were black-currant juice, (which was advised for his skin), prunes (good for the bowels), fish, eggs, chicken and fresh fruit. He never ate much meat. He liked fruit, but didn't like green vegetables. I could usually get some greens down him, however, but if he wouldn't take them after persuasion, he didn't have them.

I never rewarded him for eating foods he didn't like by giving him foods he liked, and I never used food as a reward or punishment.

His food was usually the same as ours. He first made efforts to feed himself at about eighteen months, and used to slop about a lot. I didn't bother to teach him any table-manners before he was two.

(5) *Elimination*

I began toilet-training when Peter was four months old, as I thought he might begin to get used to the idea at this age. My baby-book (*Parentcraft* by the National Association for Maternal and Child Welfare) suggested starting at two months, but I thought that was a bit too early. We didn't get any gratifying results until he was nine months old. I didn't praise him for a good performance until he was older and able to understand (about eighteen months). He was never scolded for failures. We didn't express any disgust or call him dirty.

I used to notice the time when he soiled his nappy; this was usually during the night, so I started potting him after his 10 p.m. feed. He was dry by day by about two years old, but was three before he was dry by night. We carried on with the pot until just recently, as he was frightened of the toilet-seat.

If anything, we laid more stress on motion-training. I let him sit on the pot any length of time. I used to look at the motions from a health point of view, and continued doing this till he used the toilet-seat at four years. I never made comments in Peter's presence.

He always had a tendency towards constipation, and often went two days without a motion. I only gave him a little milk of magnesia. The trouble got much worse after he was two. I must admit I was definitely worried about constipation, and took care to include prunes and lots of fresh fruit in his diet.

He only had diarrhoea once or twice; I was certainly worried, and once had to call the doctor. He told me to keep him off his food, and give him tablets for twenty-four hours.

He called motions 'poo-poo' and urine 'wee-wee'.

Even now I allow him to pass water in the street. I haven't ever told him not to mention these things in public; he himself doesn't want to mention it in front of strangers. It's not a thing we discuss freely in the family circle, and now when he wants to go he'll tell me, but won't mention it to his father.

He has seen both me and my husband in the toilet once or twice. He wouldn't understand before he was two, but now, when he comes to the toilet with me, I say 'Peter, it isn't very pleasant for you to stand here—it smells. Wouldn't it be better for you to wait downstairs?' Only recently my sister-in-law had to stop him waiting outside the lavatory till his little girl cousin came out. She told him it wasn't nice.

I treated any lapses casually. He had them when he was ill (teething, and when he had measles at one year and nine months).

He hasn't ever played with his motions; as soon as the pot was used, I whisked it away immediately.

They tell me it's good for his asthma if he belches.

(6) *Motor Development*

I used to dress him according to the weather. During the second year, he wore woollen blouses and a cardigan, cloth trousers and a woollen vest; he didn't really wear many woollies. In the summer he would wear poplin blouses, cloth trousers and an interlock vest.

His cot was certainly large enough for him to kick around in; in fact, we used it until he was four. I liked to see him waving and kicking; I looked on it as a sign of health, particularly later when he had asthma. As long as he was warm, he could have very little on.

He was strapped into his high chair until he was one year and nine months. After that he sat in an ordinary chair with a big scarf tied round him. After his meals, when he was young, he was put into his pram. I strapped him into it, and later I used shoulder-straps so that he could sit up and look around. I couldn't give any estimate of the time he spent strapped into high-chair and pram.

I sometimes carried him when he could have moved on his own, but he was rather heavy and I couldn't manage long distances. I only held him for changing and feeding at first; I thought he could get too used to it, and I had no one to help me with the house-work.

He had a play-pen from about one year to eighteen months, and stayed in it while I was busy with the housework. He didn't start to walk till eighteen months, and hadn't been crawling previously. I think it was because he had become too dependent on his play-pen; he used to walk across the house with it.

He didn't climb on the furniture till he was over two, and then I told him not to. The cupboards in the kitchen, where I kept my saucepans and so on, were forbidden to him. I kept the sideboard cupboards wedged so that he couldn't open them. I praised and encouraged him whenever he showed signs of making a new movement, such as walking, but I didn't give him any definite reward.

I got a fire-guard as soon as I saw Peter was about to walk, I had a gate made for the outside door, and arranged for a fool-proof fitting for the gas-poker. Switches weren't dangerous till later. I had a gas cooker installed instead of the double gas-ring I'd used previously, and the taps were too stiff for him to turn. He was very fond of opening the oven door, however, and I had to watch him.

I only tried to make him sit still at table; at any other time he wouldn't have taken any notice.

I never played with him in a really energetic way, as I wasn't strong enough. His father used to play with him, but I do remember that Peter disliked being lifted up high.

He was encouraged to use spoons and other implements.

(7) *Sleep*

He was an exceptionally good baby, and I had very little trouble with him about sleep.

As a baby, he slept most of the time. Then he had morning and afternoon naps; the morning nap was dropped before he was two, but the afternoon nap continued till he was three. After the 10 p.m. feed was dropped, he slept about twelve hours at night; later on he began to wake up earlier in the morning. I don't remember any more detail.

There wasn't any trouble then about going to sleep; I would just take him up to bed and leave him to go off. He gives more trouble now.

I hadn't much trouble with his waking up during the night, except when he was a young baby. Before six months, I would occasionally give him a little breast-milk, and then someone suggested glucose water. When, later on, he used to wake at 5 a.m., I would give him toys to play with.

He slept in a cot in the same room as I did. I kept on sleeping with him after he was two and a half, because it was easier for me to cope with his attacks of asthma. My husband has slept in a separate room since he developed asthma himself, on coming out of the Forces. Last year Peter was put into the third bedroom by himself.

As a baby, he wore nightdresses, as it's easier to change nappies then. He began to wear sleeping-suits after about eighteen months.

(8) *Health*

I didn't have any particular anxieties about his health during the first six months; after that I was worried about his coming into contact with any infectious illness.

He wasn't vaccinated until thirteen months, as his skin wasn't perfect. He was inoculated against diphtheria shortly afterwards, but wasn't inoculated against whooping-cough. Both times his reactions were quite normal.

He was circumcised for religious reasons.

At six weeks he developed a very slight skin rash on one side of his face—they said he had an allergy to milk generally. He had a very slight attack of chickenpox at nine months, and measles at one year and nine months. In these cases he was nursed at home; I isolated myself from the rest of the family to look after him. The asthma began when he was two and a half.

We looked to the doctor for medical advice, and I was responsible for him. I did take him to the clinic once, when he had the rash at six weeks. They advised me to put white vaseline on it, with disastrous results; I didn't go again.

We didn't have regular check-ups.

He didn't spend any time in hospital.

(9) *Physical Contacts, Masturbation, Sex-Play*

I was the only one to look after him when he was young. Occasionally, if I had any special shopping to do, I would leave him at my mother's, but that was all.

I gave him a lot of love and caresses when I picked him up. Somehow he seemed to demand a lot of affection, and still does. I used to lift him up, kiss and rock him. The affection was there all the time, but I could express my feelings more when he was older and understood.

My husband saw him in the mornings. During the first few months my husband had his tailor's workshop at home, and saw quite a lot of Peter. He used to prance round the house with him. My two brothers, my sister and my mother were all very affectionate to him.

I wouldn't have liked other people to kiss him on the mouth, but they were all too sensible to do it.

I should think baby boys and girls get about the same amount of love and kissing, but I haven't any experience of my own.

I have asked Peter to kiss other members of the family, but I think that was after he was two.

I gave his sex-organs just ordinary attention when I bathed him, but took care to powder them well. He used to call his penis his 'pisher', and now he calls it his 'willie'. He really played with himself very little, only once or twice. My feeling was that the less I paid attention to it the better. He was actually more interested in his nipples; he kept rubbing them so that they got very inflamed at one time. Now he's very curious about that sort of thing; only the other day he asked me 'Mummy, have you got a pisher?' I told him I had, so he wanted to see it. I told him it wasn't very nice for people to go round showing each other their pishers.

(10) *Clothing and Self-Exposure*

I didn't teach him to be ashamed of undressing in front of me or his father. We have very few visitors to the house, but I have never worried about undressing him in front of strangers. Why make a mystery about it?

When he was a baby, I used to say 'good boy' when he brought up his wind. I began to teach him to say 'pardon' for breaking wind, or belching, when he was about two. He was rather slow in talking (eighteen months for his first word) so I couldn't start too early. It wouldn't make any difference to these habits if he had been a girl.

We don't really undress in front of him, though he has seen me in my underclothes at times. Peter and I slept in the same room, but not in the same bed.

We had so many dresses for him that he wore them till he was about ten or eleven months. He changed into rompers then, but if he'd been a girl he would have worn dresses all the time.

(11) *Sex Distinctions*

I definitely wanted a boy, but I don't think my husband would have minded either way. As a matter of fact, though, I made a lot of dresses while I was carrying him, as I was sure I would have a girl. My husband was always talking about a girl. There were no differences in the layette; I think using different colours for boys and girls is stupid.

I used to think and talk about him as 'this baby'. Everyone else was talking about a girl—'Pamela this' and 'Pamela that'. We had names chosen for either sex before birth. My father's name in English was Paul, but his Hebrew name was Pinchas; Peter's name is Pinchas too in Hebrew, so he's really called after my father. We would have called a girl Pamela.

I was very pleased when I knew my baby was a boy. My husband was thrilled beyond imagination, and all my family was overjoyed.

The sex of the new-born baby didn't make any difference to the way he was dressed. He changed into rompers at about ten or eleven months, and by one year he hadn't any dresses at all. He didn't have much hair, but I know I cut off some of the straggly ends myself before he was two, so that his hair would be short. He never had any dolls.

I don't know of any differences in routine, discipline, or diet between baby boys and girls.

His sex didn't influence my feelings or actions in any way while I was bathing or changing him.

I don't think there's really any difference in the amount of mothering they get at this age. I have noticed, however, that my husband tends to fondle other people's little girls more than other people's little boys. It doesn't make any difference with your own child.

I used to put his nappies on double, so there wasn't any difference according to sex.

Peter has never been mistaken for a girl by anyone.

He began to stand up to pass water as soon as he was able to stand and walk alone. I think we taught him to do it. He stopped using the pot for urine a little after he was two.

He used to play in the dining-room or in the garden if the weather was suitable. Being a girl wouldn't have made any difference. I think the difference comes later, when boys themselves want to play out more than girls do. They want more freedom, so they get it.

I think little boys at this age are always hankering after their mothers. This was particularly true with Peter.

(12) Sibling Relations

This section does not apply.

(13) Relation to Parents

I was most definitely the parent mainly responsible for Peter's care.

I think my husband and I wanted a child equally.

His arrival meant quite a lot of additional expense. We didn't take out a special insurance for him.

I played with him whenever I had time, not for any definite period. Mostly this happened to be in the late afternoon, as I was less busy then. My husband didn't join in then, as he wasn't home from business. His only contact with Peter was through playing with him; he did nothing at all to help me with the work. In fact I may say that he's *not* a useful man.

I was responsible for disciplining Peter. His father spoiled him, gave him all he wanted, and would let him do absolutely anything. If anything, he tried to conceal Peter's bad behaviour from me; I certainly don't do anything of the sort with him.

I think children are capable of misbehaving when they're about three. Up to then they don't really know right from wrong.

My husband and I have definitely had disagreements about Peter, and we've had them in front of Peter. I've tried to avoid it; I know now about all this conflict being bad for his asthma, but it's difficult to prevent it entirely. My husband and I have quarrelled more since Peter's arrival than we ever did before.

I would prefer Peter to become a professional man, and I certainly hope he will achieve more than his father, both socially and otherwise. His father doesn't look so far ahead; his main interest at the moment is that Peter should get well again. I definitely hope his position in life will be better than ours.

I don't think there were any quarrels between Peter and myself at this early age; they came later after he was two.

I said I was sorry if I'd been in the wrong. His father never needed to, as he never reprimanded him in any way.

(14) *Relation to Adults other than Parents*

My family has had quite a lot to do with Peter, although none of them live with us. They're sensible enough to treat him more or less in the same way that I do. My mother, God bless her, is a very sensible woman. I didn't really expect him to behave better with them than with me.

In five years, my husband and I have had exactly two evenings out together, once to a wedding, when we had a sitter-in, and once to the pictures, when my mother-in-law stayed with Peter.

We scarcely have any people coming to visit us, but if anyone came I would bring Peter out for them to make a fuss of him. Again, I only go visiting occasionally, as I haven't any regular friend. I expect him to behave rather better then.

(15) *Possessions*

I think he first realized that things belonged to certain people when he was two and a half. He didn't really take things which weren't his; he jealously guarded his own possessions and didn't bother about other people's.

He didn't have anything much that he could understand was his own. There was a special cupboard allotted to him for his own toys, and he had his own plastic feeding dishes. I let him do whatever he liked with them.

He wasn't destructive before he was two; in fact he was the perfect little gentleman till then. Later on he started taking wheels off toys and that sort of thing. I would say 'That's not a very nice thing to do —that cost a lot'.

(16) *Speech*

You can tell the difference between their cries, but I don't know how to put it into words. If he cried when he should have been sleeping, and it sounded as though he was rebelling against sleep, I wouldn't go to him. I went if it sounded really angry, as though something was the matter. I never punished him for crying.

I very much liked to hear him babbling and trying to talk, and it was never a nuisance to me. I talked to him a great deal, but he was slow in speaking; his first word wasn't till he was eighteen months. I tried to get him to say things like 'Mama' and 'Dada'.

I showed him if I was cross with him by the expression on my face. I didn't usually try to keep him quiet. If I thought he needed something to interest him I would give him a toy to play with.

(17) *Games, Songs, Stories*

The first games we played were Pat-a-cake, Fly-away Peter, throwing balls, and, with his father, pick-a-back. We played them when we had time. I can't remember what age Peter was, but I don't think he was very young. Later he would play alone a lot, with toys, but there again not much before he was two. He had a play-pen from one year. As he didn't begin to talk before eighteen months, he couldn't really ask for us to play with him.

I would have allowed older children to play with him, but he was never very co-operative.

He was taken out in the pram by me, his father, and by my mother. I know we changed to a push-chair before he was two. We would go to the shops, occasionally on visits or to Potternewton Park. He went to Hull to visit relatives twice, once at eleven months and also for his second birthday party. He has travelled on trams, buses, and trains, which he didn't like, and in a car once or twice, which he did like.

My voice isn't good, so I didn't sing to him much. His father did occasionally, mainly nursery rhymes. There weren't any Yiddish songs. My husband isn't religious, although I am, and he doesn't bother at all about Jewish things. Jewish children now have more or less the same games and songs as ordinary children; except for their Hebrew education later there isn't much difference at all. He has picked up quite a few Yiddish expressions from my mother, however.

I never told him any stories. His father began to tell him stories, made-up, about everyday events, when he was about two, every night before going to bed.

Before two is a tender age for picture books. He had his first ones when he was about two—an alphabet book and a book of animal pictures.

We have the radio on most of the time, but we haven't a gramophone or piano.

As he got older we would go out more, but he always stuck to my apron-strings. He didn't ask to go out.

He had his own parties for his first and second birthday, and he's been to two parties held by other children living in our street. He behaved quite well.

CLINICAL REPORT

Born June 1947, at a private nursing home in Leeds.

Complaint

Referred to the Department of Psychiatry in November, 1950, by a paediatrician, with a diagnosis of 'Behaviour disorders and asthma'. Note on Clinical Condition (from paediatrician):

'This child's psychological background is very bad. He gets attacks of asthma which, I feel, are psychological in origin, also he has behaviour disorders of various kinds'.

Mother's Account of Problem (given at first interview):
Asthmatic attacks began at age of two and a half years, and since have occurred regularly but with varying severity. During the attack he becomes pallid, lifeless, and has a rapid pulse. Some of the spasms are painful and leave him exhausted. He has great difficulty in breathing and will say 'Mummy help me with my breath'. If given an antispasmodic, he sleeps and is recovering by the time he wakes, but is left lifeless and listless for a day or two.

Behaviour disorders

(*a*) Inclined to spit if he did not get his own way.
(*b*) Becomes very excited if thwarted.
(*c*) Stubborn.
(*d*) Bossy with other children. Suspicious that they want to steal his toys.

S   267

Fears

When (*a*) left alone
    (*b*) demands light in bedroom and someone to stay with him till he sleeps
    (*c*) occasional enuresis till three years
    (*d*) nightmares began at three years; says there are spiders on his pillow
    (*e*) used to have (from two years) marked 'startle' reaction, i.e. head hidden with arm.

Family History

Mother—aged 42.

A neatly dressed, prim woman, who appeared depressed and lacking in spontaneity, when first seen at the clinic. She has a careful, over-refined way of speaking. She was fussy, nervous and anxiously expecting trouble, in her attitude towards Peter.

She is of Jewish origin, and is one of a family of seven. She describes great inter-sibling affection and sympathy. She still has a close relationship with her mother, who lives in Leeds and is not in good health. Her mother is being looked after by two unmarried sons 'who are as good as women to her'.

Mrs. R.'s health has 'never been good'. She has a 'bad back', and thought she had a hernia recently which, on examination, proved to be nothing. A sprained ankle takes her to hospital. She has, however, had attacks of phlebitis. When Peter was a baby she was unable to play rowdy games with him.

When breast-feeding the baby she felt weak and faint, but nevertheless describes it as a wonderful experience. When she put him down after a feed, and more especially after she had weaned him, she felt that her 'arms were empty'.

She has great social ambitions which she cannot satisfy. When among those whom she considers her inferiors, she puts on a genteel manner and cuts herself off from them. On the other hand, when she attended functions of a local Jewish society run by wealthy and, from her point of view, socially 'high class' people, she felt unable to compete at such levels of hospitality. She is therefore not at home with either group, and she herself remarks that she has very few friends.

Father—aged 49, a tailor by trade.

Born in England of a Russian Jewish family. He has not actually been seen by anyone at the clinic.

His father emigrated from Russia to England with his first wife, who died in childbirth. Her sister, then aged 16 years, was sent over to look after the child, and a year later married Mr. R.'s father.

She had nine children, of whom Mr. R. was the eldest, and all of whom are alive. She was not very intelligent, according to Mrs. R., and never learned to speak English well. Nor had she much time for her children, so that Mr. R. felt neglected. In contrast, Mrs. R.'s family 'would all suffer if she hurt her little finger', but Mr. R.'s family were hard towards each other.

Mr. R. is said to have had a talent for painting and wanted to make it his career. His schoolmaster offered to pay for two years' tuition at an art school, but his wages were needed at home and he was not allowed to accept this offer. He is therefore very anxious that Peter should not be deprived, and worries incessantly about whether his diet is correct or whether he is happy. Mrs. R. thinks he spoils Peter.

He developed asthma while serving in His Majesty's Forces. He is still having attacks, which are relieved by a nasal inhalant, and is often up during the night.

When asked whether Mr. R. would come to the clinic, Mrs. R. became anxious and asked whether he would be told what she had said. He is rather antagonistic to the idea of Peter's attending the clinic, as he feels that there is a stigma attached to it. She would like him to attend, provided the staff did not discuss family differences if he brought them up.

Relationship between Father and Mother

Mrs. R. says that the marriage was a happy one before her husband went away to the armed forces. After the baby was born on his return, she became very 'disappointed' in her husband. He speaks, she feels, in an uneducated way, and she is upset when Peter imitates him. Mr. R. accuses her of being unsympathetic when Peter has an attack of asthma. They have not slept together since the asthma began.

Mrs. R. makes repeated references to her husband's moroseness and bad manners. She is afraid to go on holiday with him, in case he will 'show her up' by swearing and making scenes. As he is frequently moody and depressed, she considers that he is no company for her.

Mrs. R. is strictly orthodox in religion, and is very particular about observance of rites, but her husband does not bother. This is regarded by her as another example of the slackness of his family.

Discussing marital difficulties, she blushed, stammered and said that, if it had not been for Peter, the marriage would have broken up by mutual consent. She feels discouraged about the future and wonders what she will do when Peter no longer needs so much attention.

Just prior to referral there had been acute friction between them over Mr. R.'s relatives. Since returning from the war, Mr. R. and a brother set up a tailoring firm, the latter looking after the business side. Mrs. R. feels her husband is imposed upon by his brother, and is contemptuous because he does not demand his rights.

This brother and his wife live next door, and recently they suggested that Mrs. R. should take her father-in-law to live with her. On the grounds that he has four daughters alive, Mrs. R. declined, with the result that she was ostracized. Rather defensively, she takes the line that she has nothing in common with them anyway, as they are rough and ill-spoken. The partnership between the brothers has now been dissolved and tension is diminishing.

Pregnancy and Birth of Peter

Marriage had lasted fifteen years before conception took place. Her doctor had told her that she 'needed stretching' before she could conceive, but she did not have this done. Her husband served in the Forces during the war and it was on his return that she became pregnant, at the age of 37, and was granted her passionate wish.

Mother felt very well during pregnancy and was not afraid of the confinement, though she engaged a private doctor and booked a place in a nursing home. As the doctor was due to go on holiday, and wanted to get the birth over before she went, Mrs. R. was taken into the nursing home and an induction performed. There was a placenta praevia, and an episiotomy was also done. She does not remember much about it because she was anaesthetized, but she considers that she had a bad time, and alleges a certain amount of medical incompetence.

The baby was bruised about the head as a result of instrumental delivery.

Development of the Child

Birth-weight 9 lb., diminishing to 8 lb. 12 oz. in the first few days. Birth-weight plus 2 oz. regained in three weeks.

Feeding

Peter was breast-fed, at first at fixed intervals, but later on a slightly more flexible schedule.

Solids were introduced at four and a half months, the first one being a proprietary cereal food.

Weaning was very sudden, at six months, when Mrs. R. developed septic tonsillitis. According to her statements, 'he didn't seem to miss the breast at all'. Thumb-sucking began at nine months, and continued to eighteen months. His mother did not like to see it, but, on her doctor's advice, did not do anything to stop the habit.

There were no real feeding difficulties for the first two years. At the age of referral (three years five months), his appetite was normally fairly good, but poor when he was having attacks of asthma. He could sit at table, a little uncomfortably, and feed himself well. He disliked green vegetables and did not eat a great deal of meat. No stomach upsets have been reported.

Elimination

Toilet-training began at four months; the baby-book had suggested two months, but Mrs. R. thought that was a little too soon. Her attitude was lenient, and there was no question of scolding him or expressing disgust at failures. He was dry by day at two years two months, and by night at three years two months, except when he was having attacks of asthma. He gave up using the pot for urine at about two years, but refused to pass a motion into the lavatory until he was four years old.

General Development

First tooth at six months. Others followed quickly.
Walked (without preliminary crawling stage) at eighteen months.
Fed himself from eighteen months.
First two words at eighteen months.

Illnesses, operations, accidents

Eight days—ritual circumcision.
Six weeks to nine months—eczema.
Nine months—very slight chickenpox.
One year nine months—measles.
Two years six months—asthma.
Two years eleven months—fell down steps and bruised nose. Cried a great deal at this.

Psychologist's Report

Peter was tested twice, once at referral, when aged three years five months, and again, in his mother's presence, when he was four years seven months.

First Testing

'*Behaviour.* Negativistic attitude, tending to grumble in a whining voice saying "I can't do it, no I don't want to, what shall we do now" etc. His eyes did appear watery on one or two occasions but he did not cry. He was more co-operative on the second interview and it was then observed that his uncooperative moods and negativistic attitude appeared when a task was actually too difficult for him. On one or two occasions he did attempt a difficult task, after much grumbling. He did not, however, try for long.

Peter is ambidexterous. While drawing he was observed to change the pencil from one hand to the other according to whether he wanted to put a line more on the right, or left-hand side, of the drawing.

He shows perseveration in drawing, perhaps too much considering that he showed little power of concentration on various tasks such as those occurring in the Merrill Palmer and Binet tests.

He could not be made to draw a man but he would say "Yes", and draw a lorry and say a "lorry-man" or just "lorry".

Tests given:

Merrill Palmer. Approximate mental age three years.
    This result cannot be considered either reliable or valid since testing conditions were not satisfactory.

Binet L.[1] I.Q. 112. Bright level. M.A. three years ten months.
This intellectual level may not be considered a causal factor in this child's reported behaviour problems.'

Second Testing (after about a year's treatment).

'*General Behaviour.* Mother took Peter's layers of clothes off and warned me that he had had an attack before coming and that consequently he would probably not co-operate. All this was in the child's hearing. Mother encouraged him to go along with me before I had made any approaches to Peter and he refused to come. He was less negativistic when assured of Mother's presence and when a joke and a sweet had cleared the air. Nevertheless he repeated "I don't know" liberally during the test; he said this when in fact he performed with accuracy and speed, as on the Wallin Peg Boards[2]. He would open his eyes when told to keep them closed. He kissed his mother three times during the test, each time continuing with the task in hand later.

Results. Peter's Mental Age as calculated on this test is three years eleven months, so that his intelligence level is nearly one standard deviation below the mean of his chronological age (four years seven months). He may be said therefore to be of low average intelligence according to these results.

However, there were factors in the test situation which may make these results unreliable. The chief one is the presence of Mrs. R. She interrupted rarely but significantly: she would encourage him by comparing his performance with that of a little friend of his. The fact that on these occasions he would always try harder does not invalidate the theory that her presence was

[1]Revised Stanford Binet Intelligence Scale, Form L.
[2]Item in the Merrill Palmer Intelligence Scale for Children.

disturbing in general. She reminded him at all times to say "please" and "thank you". He did say "goodbye" finally, his face in Mother's skirts.

Test behaviour. Would start with enthusiasm but tended to give up easily particularly on the Sequin Form Board[1]. On each trial at least one block was left partly fitted. He refused to do the buttons and was not able to undo his own buttons. He was distractable on the Decroly Matching Games[2]; he would set out with a piece in his hand and during the search for its partner would start to match another one.

Goodenough Man Drawing.[3] Although his man had two pairs of arms and a box "cos to sleep in" it suggests a mental age of about five years. This would tend to confirm the opinion that the Merrill-Palmer result may be an underestimate of his true abilities; or it may reflect a specific talent for drawing.'

Peter's Personality

Peter is definitely a 'mummy's boy' and is very anxious when she leaves him. When Mrs. R. was seeing a new interviewer, whom he had met before, he was very reluctant to let her go, refused to recognize the interviewer, and vowed he would '*never* know her'. This attitude was not improved by his mother's hesitation and obvious desire to keep him with her, or by her remark, at the end of the interview that 'we've been talking about you, Peter'.

He is a repressed child and inhibited in many ways. Despite outbursts of temper tantrums in public and elsewhere, he is generally quiet, timid and docile.

With other children, his initial reaction is one of great timidity, and on the whole he has very little contact with them. He feels towards them a great deal of resentment of a sullen kind.

His mood upsets are probably expressed in his asthma, but at times he has behaved very emotionally, as if wishing to shame his mother in public.

Curiosity about Sex

At first, when Peter asked where he came from, his mother told him he had been bought. When he was about four and a half years, she told him that he had grown inside her, which he accepted without comment.

He is interested in his 'pisher' (the term he uses for his penis) and wants to know if he was born with it. He has also asked his mother

---

[1, 2, 3] Items in the Merrill Palmer Intelligence Scale for Children.

if she had a 'pisher', to which she replied 'Of course'. To his demand to be shown *her* pisher, she answered 'Now that's not very nice, Peter. We don't go around showing each other our pishers'. He comments on her breasts, inquiring why he has none.

Housing

The R.s live in a Victorian terrace house in a predominantly Jewish area of Leeds. The house has three bedrooms, a living-room, kitchen and bathroom.

They are on terms of tension with both next-door neighbours: one, the brother-in-law and his wife, who, in addition to other family grievances, arouse Mrs. R.'s envy by having much superior furniture; and the other, a paranoid old lady with whom there are perpetual quarrels.

2. MICHAEL

A boy of similar background to Peter's

INTRODUCTION

In finding a normal parallel for the case of Peter R., it was felt that one of the important criteria should be the Orthodox Jewish background of the mother. We were introduced to the P. family through a religious Zionist organization in Leeds, to whom we had explained the purpose of this study. Mrs. P. and her son Michael were described by them as 'normal, charming people'.

Family History

Mother. The mother is an extremely neat, pretty woman, who looks much less than her thirty-seven years. She is of small build, quick in her movements and tends to speak rapidly and emphatically. At first her attitude was polite and aloof, but in the course of the interviews she became much more friendly, and said she had really enjoyed answering the questionnaire.

She herself was born in Leeds, of an East European immigrant family. One of the youngest of eleven children, she has maintained contact with them all and with a rapidly increasing number of nieces and nephews. The whole family is extremely orthodox in its religious beliefs and practices, and the younger generation maintains this tradition; one nephew was said to associate only with rabbis, and another, at present in Israel, was one of the leaders of the religious youth movement in this country. Mrs. P., since her marriage to a less orthodox man, has become rather more lax, but her standards are still high compared with the relatively unobservant Leeds Jewish Community.

Neither of her parents is alive now.

Her life at home seems to have been rather a sheltered one, and she was not very well-instructed in the 'facts of life'. She comments on her ignorance of sex when she was first married, and it is interesting to note that after ten and a half years of married life she had no idea that labour could be painful or last longer than an hour or so.

Father. At 43, the father is a stout, comfortable-looking man, who does everything in a leisurely way. He is in the furniture business and manages to be reasonably prosperous.

He was also born in Leeds of an East European immigrant family, though his background is much less orthodox than that of his wife. He is one of four children.

His mother is still alive, and, as will be seen from the questionnaire answers, she has quite often expressed her views on Michael's upbringing. She feels that Mrs. P.'s ideas on baby care were unnecessarily strict—for example, only fondling the child at appointed times and not letting him sleep in the parents' room. She was responsible for ensuring that Michael was breast-fed, at a time when the family doctor was saying that bottle-feeding was just as good and would give Mrs. P. more freedom.

Marriage. The marriage took place, with the blessing of both families, in 1936. It is on the whole a successful one, though Mr. P. thinks his wife is inclined to fuss too much and there is a certain amount of mild bickering.

After Michael's birth, marital intercourse was not resumed for a year. According to Mrs. P., this was due to fear of another pregnancy.

Birth of Michael. Although neither of his parents at any time practised contraception, Michael was not born till ten and a half years after their marriage. They sought advice on their sterility, but the doctor could not find signs of any abnormality in either partner. Mrs. P. was very depressed about it, and could hardly bear to be alone in the house at one time. Her pregnancy was received by them both with incredulous joy.

Labour was long and difficult, and after it had gone on for three days she was transferred from the private nursing home to the Leeds Maternity Hospital for a Caesarean section. She seems to have been completely unprepared for any difficulty and it was not long before she lost control. She expresses surprise that she should have taken it so badly, as she is normally 'hard rather than soft'. The experience made such a profound impression on her that, in spite of her years of longing for a baby, she absolutely refused to see him for three days after the birth. 'I didn't want to own him'. Her attitude, which was unaffected by her husband's pleading, broke down suddenly when she overheard the nurses saying 'Any volunteers for feeding Baby P.?' She fed him, and after that could not do too much for him. After three weeks at the maternity hospital she returned to her nursing home for another three weeks, then spent a fortnight learning how to look after the baby at her sister-in-law's, and returned home when Michael was eight weeks old.

Upbringing. The details of Michael's upbringing for the first two years are given, in his mother's own words, in the following account.

On the whole it was a fairly strict one; feeding and fondling took place at definite and regular intervals, and great stress was laid on toilet-training. This began at six weeks and achieved complete success—dryness by day and night—at one year eleven months. Throughout the whole account, it is clear that Mrs. P. feels great revulsion against the process of excretion and would like to think the alimentary canal ended at the mouth. Michael's playing with his penis also worries her a great deal, though she says she tries not to show it.

Michael's Personality and Behaviour at nearly Six Years

Michael, who is now nearly six, is a remarkably attractive young boy with an easy, casual manner. He is very quick, lively and energetic.

He has been at the local primary school now for nearly a year, being slightly older than Peter R. There he is making very fast progress, so much so that his teacher visited the home to request them not to give him private coaching, which they had never done. He, in company with most of his class-mates, is closely attached to his teacher, a young attractive girl who treats each boy as an individual. He is upset at the thought of moving into a higher class next year, as he does not want to leave her.

Before his present school, he attended a nursery school for two years.

Difficulties are now beginning to arise between mother and son. He claims that she is 'trying to make a cissy of him'. Mrs. P. is highly critical of the other mothers in the neighbourhood, who allow their children to wear scanty clothing, do not insist on a regular bed-time, and often do not bother where their offspring are from one hour to the next. Michael resents having to do things that the other boys are not bothered with, especially as his playmates are given to chanting, in an amused tone, 'Michael has to go in, Michael has to go in'. In spite of this difficulty, he gets on extremely well with the neighbourhood children, both of his own age and older, both Jewish and non-Jewish. In their soldier games, he holds the rank of field-marshal, and his influence was great enough to get a little girl of four, who would normally have been shunned, accepted as an A.T.S. contingent. There is a certain amount of fighting among the boys, which, to their great disgust, Mrs. P. takes seriously and tries to stop. Recently, she has made her presence felt at the school, where she requested the teacher to stop his mid-morning milk as it blunted his appetite for lunch. He is now, against his will, the only boy in his form who does not have milk.

He responds to these frustrations, which so often take place in

277

front of his companions, by terrific outbreaks of temper. One day, while he was walking to school with a friend, Mrs. P. followed after him with a mackintosh. He told her that the other boys didn't wear them, but she nevertheless insisted, so he stamped and screamed and threw the mackintosh down in the road. She was extremely hurt by this behaviour and resolved to be very cold to him when he returned home; but his cheerful friendliness quickly melted her. Apparently he never has outbreaks of temper at school, but dislikes frustration in the tasks he sets himself and is apt to blame other people for his failure in anything. Mrs. P. says that no sooner has he lost his temper than he is perfectly normal again, smiles and waves at her, and runs out to play leaving her to cope with her own reactions. Mr. P. does not take any of this very seriously, and merely points out that several members of Mrs. P.'s family have bad tempers.

A more unusual problem is presented by his extreme fastidiousness about feeding and going to the toilet. This has only developed very recently, to his mother's great surprise. He will not eat anything that has been touched by another person, even his mother, and he is reluctant to use a toilet that someone else might have used. Mrs. P. finds his attitude inconsistent, as he does not care how dirty he gets, will eat with filthy hands, and does not mind touching food intended for other people. She claims that nothing she has done or said could be in any way responsible for this behaviour.

It will therefore be seen that this 'normal child' and his mother do not present a completely harmonious picture.

Development

First tooth, six and a half months.
Crawled, ten months.
Stood, one year and one month.
Walked, one year and two months.
Said 'Dada', seven months.
Said 'Mama', one year.
At two years he could manage phrases like 'Some more tea'.

Housing

A small semi-detached, three-bedroomed house in a residential area of Leeds. There are parks and woods nearby, and a stream at the bottom of the garden. A large number of Jewish people live in the district.

The interior is in very good condition, freshly decorated and well-kept. The father has made a great deal of the furniture and fittings himself.

*   *   *   *   *

(This account, by Michael's mother, Mrs. P., was compiled from her answers to the Leeds Questionaire.)

UPBRINGING FOR THE FIRST TWO YEARS

(1) *Mother's Attitude towards having Children*

I first found out that I could have children when I was about fifteen or sixteen. I didn't know many of the details, and I can't remember now how I found out, or from whom. I was one of a family of eleven, so my mother didn't have much opportunity to give us individual attention or instruction. When I got married I was very naïve about these things.

We tried to have a child right from the very beginning of our marriage, but we didn't succeed for ten and a half years. Both of us went to the doctor when we realized there might be something wrong, but apparently we were completely normal and he couldn't give us any explanation of our childlessness. I was advised to rest more, relax and take things easy.

I was very surprised indeed when I found I was pregnant, and my first feeling was one of incredulity—I was too overjoyed to think it was true. Needless to say I was very pleased, and so was my husband, who adores children. My father had died a year before I became pregnant, and my mother became very ill three months after his death, as though she just couldn't get on without him. Nevertheless she was thrilled at the idea of my having a baby.

I would most definitely have been worried if there had been no possibility of my having children. In fact, that was the way it seemed to be, and I got so depressed over it that I couldn't bear to stay in the house. I had to go out all the time to try and forget myself and my disappointment.

I wouldn't have adopted a child, however. In a family like mine there's no need for anyone to be without a child: I could always 'borrow' one to look after for a while, and I would have spent my life being a good 'Auntie'.

If income and health allowed it, I would like to have two children.

The drawback about having children is childbirth. I had a very bad delivery and it took me three months to get over the shock of it. When I came home afterwards I said to my husband 'We'll sleep in separate rooms after this'. He didn't take me seriously! Now I would say that you certainly go through it at the time, but later you get over it and forget it.

I had to have a Caesarean in the end, as I was rather small.

(2) *Mother's Experiences during Pregnancy*

While I was carrying Michael I never felt better in my whole life. The only trouble was during the first month. We were on holiday at

279

the seaside and I thought it was the seaweed that made me feel sick on and off. My sister, who was with us and herself pregnant at the time, said 'Wouldn't it be funny, Lee, if you were pregnant as well?' I laughed at her at the time, but in the end she turned out to be right.

As I said before, I was very naïve about the 'facts of life' and I didn't know much about having a baby. My sister told me there was nothing to be scared of. I just thought it would be like having a period pain and I'd no idea at all how long it would take. I thought it was just a matter of a few hours.

I was embarrassed by my size at first; I looked so big that I thought I was going to have twins. After a while I got used to it. Michael wasn't a very active baby while I was carrying him.

I didn't do any less housework during this time, but I did take a rest after dinner and didn't go into town regularly as I had done before. I avoided stretching or anything like that. I took care to eat more regularly and carefully—before I'd just taken my meal to suit myself and sometimes would content myself with a sandwich or something like that. Now I felt I was responsible for someone else as well. I had some maternity clothes made for me and must say I looked very trim. I think I took more care of myself and my appearance during that time than ever before or since.

The main thing I avoided was stretching. I took lots of oranges, because a book I read—a rather unusual one by one of those nature-cure people—said they would make for an easy confinement. According to the woman who wrote it, labour is the easiest thing in the world provided you follow her diet and so on.

No one else had to make any changes in behaviour because of my pregnancy.

The doctor who was looking after me gave me the details of the baby's weight as we went along, and advised me to diet so that he shouldn't be a big baby.

I used to read the women's magazines, especially the *Women's Pictorial*. At the nursing home they didn't teach me a thing about looking after babies. It was six weeks before I even saw him undressed. After I came home my sister-in-law showed me how to do everything.

(3) *Birth*

I thought childbirth was an easy thing, and that was the way my family let me look on it. I soon got a surprise.

I'd booked at a private nursing home for the confinement, and between you and me they were very bad; I understand they've since had to close down. After I'd been in labour for three days, they realized things weren't quite as they should be, and I was whisked off to hospital. They, on the other hand, were simply marvellous.

I had injections for the first part of the confinement at the nursing home, and for the Caesarean I had complete anaesthesia. I wasn't conscious when the baby arrived and I didn't hear him cry for the first time.

The hospital specialist was there at the operation, and I should think there were nurses as well. I didn't mind who was or who wasn't there.

I thought childbirth was a terrible experience. My husband tells me that I was making a terrible to-do before I left for the nursing home, and when I got there the matron said 'For heaven's sake be quiet, Mrs. P., or you'll wake everyone in the road'. I felt so dreadful about it that I just refused to see Michael for the first three days. My husband kept on saying: 'When are you going to see him, Lee?'—but I just didn't want to.

It was all quite a big expense to us. It was that very expensive time just after the war.

My father died a year before Michael was born, and we've always felt that I had to wait for a child so I could give him my father's name. It's a strange thing, too, but Michael now seems to have a lot of my father's characteristics, so that you could almost think of him as being a reincarnation—if you believe in that sort of thing.

Michael was as ugly as he could be when he was born, but his father thought he was just wonderful.

He wasn't christened, but circumcised, as we are Jews.

It was about two months before I recovered properly from the confinement.

(4) *Feeding*

I didn't feed Michael till three days after he was born. As I said before, I refused to see him, but on the third day I overheard the nurses talking: 'Any volunteers for feeding Baby P. today?' When I heard that I knew that I must own him, so I called out 'Yes, me'.

He was breast-fed. At the hospital you don't get the choice; they make you do it. They said I had sufficient for him. I had a cracked nipple after a while, for which they gave me rather painful electrical treatment. When I got home, my own doctor didn't care whether I breast or bottle-fed him, but my mother-in-law assured me that breast-feeding would be much better for Michael. By then I loved him so much that I'd have done anything for him.

I found nursing was a painful experience for me. My own doctor told me 'If you put him on the bottle you'll be able to have your freedom', but in the end I didn't take any notice of that.

Michael was a good feeder, in fact he was very good generally. I fed him in my arms, in the usual way. Feeding was by the clock, and if he cried before time was up I would nurse him a little but not feed him. If he was asleep when feeding-time came round I would wake him up. I think this way is more convenient for getting them into routine and for the household as well.

He never refused food and he never stopped feeding before he'd taken what he needed. I never had too little milk.

Intercourse was restricted for almost a year after Michael was born.

I began to wean him gradually at eight and a half months. He had two good teeth by then, so I thought it was time. I certainly never tried to disgust him with the breast. My neighbour helped me by feeding him when I was out of the room.

I gave him a rusk to chew when he was about five or six months old, but he threw it away. He had a little silver ornament but didn't put it in his mouth much. I never gave him a dummy.

There was no thumb-sucking, but he has always sucked his tongue since he was a tiny baby. He does it now whenever he's concentrating particularly hard on something.

I started to introduce solids at four and a half months, by spoon; the first was egg, and then, I think, sieved grated apple. We fed him alone, in his own room. Mealtimes were regular. I didn't worry if he refused food at one meal. I took the attitude that what he didn't have at one meal he would have at the next. He was never a poor eater.

At other people's houses he has over-eaten once or twice. I gave him milk of magnesia if I thought he'd had too much.

Good foods, I thought, were vegetables, fruit and soups; bad were sauces, vinegar and condiments ,and anything with too much flavouring. He doesn't particularly like meat, chicken or very sweet things.

I didn't try to bribe him to eat things he didn't like by offering things he did like, and I didn't use food as a reward or punishment in other cases.

Before he was one year old, his food was quite different from ours; during the second year it was more or less the same, except that he didn't have meat till he was nearly two.

He started using a spoon at ten months. The book said that mess didn't matter; what they don't eat with the spoon they eat with their fingers. I didn't attempt to teach any table manners at this age.

(5) *Elimination*

I began toilet-training him when we returned home six weeks after his birth. This was what I'd been taught to do at the hospital; as I said before, the nursing home didn't give me any instruction. I was lucky with him until he began to realize what it was all about, and then I wasn't lucky. At one year and six months he was still in nappies, but by one year and eleven months he was dry by day and by night. I put him into a bed then.

I used to praise him when he managed a good performance. I began telling him off for wetting and soiling after he'd started walking, at about one year and three months. There isn't much point in doing that until they can understand. At that age we began to show disgust about urine and faeces.

He was potted before and after feeds. I didn't lift him at night, because I thought sleep was more important than cleanliness.

I think the average child should be dry by day and night at about two.

I think bowel-training is much easier than bladder-training, but I didn't feel that one was more important than the other.

I would only allow him to sit for five to ten minutes on the pot.

I used to examine what he'd done till he was about three, but I never made any comments to him.

He never had any constipation, and the only time he had diarrhoea was after eating soft fruit. It has never agreed with me, either, and now we neither of us eat soft fruit. I didn't really have to bother with any special preventives or remedies.

He used to say 'mo-mo' before motions and 'wee' for urine. This was all right at first, but I couldn't stand it really, and taught him to say 'going to the toilet' as soon as he could talk. I think that's the only really nice word for it; you get people saying such blunt and crude things like 'going to the lavatory' and I don't like it.

I allowed him to 'wee' in the street, but he had to wait for motions.

I didn't make a particular point of teaching him not to talk about these things in public, and now he's far too outspoken. He will be out playing with his friends, sometimes even with little girls, and he'll call to them 'Wait for me—I've just got to go to the toilet'.

We never let him see us in the toilet; my husband doesn't even allow him in the bathroom while he's shaving.

He never had any lapses after he was trained, except once at the nursery school after he was three.

He *never* did anything like playing with his motions.

As soon as he could talk, I taught him to say 'excuse me' if he did anything rude.

(6) *Motor Development*

As soon as he could crawl, he wore buster-rompers round the house.

He had an average-size cot that my husband made for him, so he had plenty of room to kick around in it. I liked to see him waving and kicking as much as he wanted, and he never had much on in the way of clothes.

We strapped him into his chair for meals when he got more energetic. This was just for meals, or sometimes between meals when I had to go out of the room to fetch something. At about one year, he was strapped into his pram when we went out.

I very often carried him when he could really walk himself, to save time.

He had a play-pen from about seven months to one year, but only spent about half an hour in it each day.

He was *not* allowed to climb on the furniture. I didn't allow him to go on the stairs after he'd had two falls there—one at about six months and the other at one year and two months.

When he made a new movement, I told him I was pleased and he was a clever boy. We taught him to walk and to climb up the stairs.

We always told him fires were hot, and he's never gone near them, so we haven't needed a guard. In our house you can't touch the switches. He had an electric shock when he was eighteen months at a friend's house. Here the plugs are shock-proof.

It wasn't necessary to make him sit still before he was two. I do know it's bad for him now to get over-excited, so I try to get him to sit still for a time.

Both my husband and I used to play energetic games on the floor with him—like playing elephants.

We encouraged him to use spoons and other implements.

(7) *Sleep*

He's always loved his sleep. Till he was two, he used to have naps both in the morning and the afternoon, usually about one and a half hours in each case.

Before he went to sleep, we used to sing and tell him little stories about ourselves. This started when he was a few weeks old. After six months, we began to sing him nursery-rhyme songs. He never woke up in the middle of the night.

He slept in a cot in a room by himself right from the very start. My mother-in-law said 'How can you be so cruel—he might call you and you wouldn't know.'

Till eighteen months he wore nightdresses (with a vest in winter). Then he began to wear pyjamas.

(8) *Health*

He was a normal healthy child. I hadn't seen any children that weren't, so I didn't worry about any diseases in his case. I thought teething might cause a little trouble.

He was vaccinated and immunized against diphtheria, but we didn't bother about whooping-cough.

He was circumcised for religious reasons. He reacted in the usual way, yelling and then going to sleep.

He never had any illnesses. I would go to the doctor if anything were wrong. I didn't go to a clinic or have regular check-ups.

(9) *Physical Contacts, Masturbation, Sex-Play*

The only person, besides myself, who looked after him during the first two years, was my sister-in-law. This was just for a fortnight after I came out of the nursing home, while I was learning how to look after him.

Michael got a lot of loving, but it was at the proper times, before and after feeds, and after his bath-time. My mother-in-law thought you should love babies when you feel like it, and never mind what time it is. I don't know. I did what I thought was right, but different people say different things, don't they?

I think the amount of loving he got was more or less the same throughout the first two years.

Only the members of our two families came into really close contact with him. I think our families, especially my husband's, tend to spoil him.

I didn't let other people handle him when he was very young, even at my mother-in-law's. Later, other people were allowed to play with him, but not to kiss him. I have a horror that other people might kiss him, and certainly don't encourage him to kiss others.

My family doesn't make any difference between boys and girls as far as kissing is concerned, but my mother-in-law fusses much more over boys.

When I bathed him, I just treated his genitals normally. He called his penis his 'little Johnnie'. I think other children play with their sex organs, but when I compare him with his friend Neville, who is so modest, I do wonder whether Michael is really just the same as others. Now I sometimes come into the bathroom and find him stroking his penis, saying 'Poor little thing. Poor little thing—it's so hot'. Sometimes I try to ignore it and sometimes I say 'Michael, you are soft'. My husband tells me to think nothing of it.

(10) *Clothing and Self-Exposure*

I didn't exactly teach Michael to be ashamed of being naked, but as soon as he could understand I would tell him that little children don't go around without any clothes on.

At about three months I began to correct him for breaking wind, and when he was old enough to speak I taught him to say "Cuse me'.

I used to say 'good boy' when he brought his wind *up* as a baby. I think in this sort of thing I would have been more particular with a girl—I'm sure, for example, that I would never have let a girl 'wee' in public.

My husband and I never undressed or washed in front of Michael. I could never see any sense in it.

He had a room to himself right from the start.

He wore a romper right from the beginning, but at first it was un-closed between his legs. At nine months he changed into a buster-romper. This is because he's a boy.

(11) *Sex Distinctions*

I didn't mind what sex my child was, as long as it was healthy. I prepared for either in the layette. Everything was white; there was none of that silly nonsense about pink or blue things. In Michael's day the chamber-pots weren't different for boys and girls, but I gather they are now. Girls wear bonnets and boys pixie hoods, but those are the only differences I know in clothing for the newly-born.

I thought of the baby as 'it' while I was carrying him. I knew that any boy would be called by my father's Hebrew name, but I didn't choose English names for either sex before the birth.

As I've said before, I refused to see the baby for three days after he was born, and I had no reactions at all to his sex. My husband and both our families were very pleased and thrilled.

I started trimming his hair at about six months, to keep it short like a boy's, and it was first cut at a barber's when he was two.

His sex didn't make any difference to the toys he got during the first six months. He had little dolls, and I don't know whether this has anything to do with it, but he loves babies now and is always looking into prams.

I don't know of any differences in routine for boys and girls.

His sex didn't make me feel any different while I was bathing or changing him. It didn't affect the amount of mothering he got.

Nappies are fixed in the same way for boys and girls.

Michael was mistaken once or twice for a girl, at the time when he had all his hair on. I wasn't upset, because it was only occasionally and by people who, in my opinion, didn't matter.

I don't know of any differences in diet, toilet-training or discipline between baby boys and girls, except of course that little boys have to learn to stand to pass water. We taught Michael to do this at about eighteen months. He continued to use the pot till he was three. I think that girls are probably easier to train than boys.

When Michael had picture-books they were usually about soldiers, trains and engines; girls usually read things about Dollie this and

Dollie that. As for games, boys like buckets, spades and everything dirty, but little girls don't like to get dirty. There isn't any difference in the freedom they're allowed till school age.

There was no difference in Michael's preference for me or my husband.

(12) *Sibling Relations*

Michael is the only child.

(13) *Relation to Parents*

With the exception of one fortnight at my sister-in-law's, I have always been mainly responsible for looking after Michael.

Both my husband and I wanted a child equally.

His coming made a great difference to family spending. We took an insurance policy out in my name, because the company wouldn't do it in Michael's own name.

The regular times for playing with him were before and after his feeds and after his bath. Both my husband and I used to join in.

My husband used to like to massage Michael after his bath, and would play with him, nurse and soothe him. He would change his nappies if I happened to be out, but never fed or bathed him.

We are both responsible for discipline, but I think my husband was if anything rather stricter than I was. He made up for it by being over-generous in giving things. Anyhow, I would tell Michael to 'wait till your father comes home' and he would be very quiet after that. We neither of us attempted to conceal Michael's bad behaviour from each other. Sometimes we disagree about discipline—though I would never call it quarrelling—but we try not to do it in front of Michael.

I think children are capable of misbehaving as soon as they can talk and understand what you say; at about two, I should imagine.

I would really like Michael to follow his own bent in life. His father is very anxious that he should have a marvellous education, and is determined to make him work hard and take full advantage of it. He wishes he had taken more notice of his own parents and worked harder when he was at school. Michael now says he would like to be a professional man. We hope his place in life will be better than ours.

We never had what you'd call quarrels before Michael was two.

If my husband and I were ever in the wrong we would admit it quite willingly.

(14) *Relation to Adults other than Parents*

My sister-in-law, for the fortnight we stayed with her after coming out of the nursing home, was the only person who had a great deal to do with him before he was two.

287

We had a sitter-in for him till he was nearly two. I wouldn't want him to wake up and find a stranger there, so either my husband or I always stayed in with him.

I know there are different schools of thought about bringing babies down when there are visitors. We only did it once, when he was six weeks old, and it never happened again. As a matter of fact, he only came into the dining-room when his play-pen was there.

I didn't take him visiting often, though he went to Sheffield quite a few times to see my sister. On these occasions I expected him to behave in his usual way.

(15) *Possessions*

I think he first became aware of things belonging to certain people when he was about a year old. If he took things that weren't his, I punished him by smacking his hand. I was more annoyed if he snatched, and didn't like it even if the thing was his own.

His toys, eating and toilet-things were his very own. He had to be careful with them. At first, if he tried to damage something, I would tell him not to; if he did it again, I would smack him. On the whole he wasn't very destructive, however.

(16) *Speech*

He didn't cry a lot when he was young. Sometimes I could ignore it, and it would pass into singing after a while. I usually went to him, as he didn't do it often and usually had some good reason. I never punished him for crying.

I liked to hear him babbling and trying to talk, and never found it a nuisance. I talked to him a great deal and encouraged him to answer me.

In those days, if I was annoyed with him, I'd say 'I'm cross with you.' Now, I say 'You're going back where you came from'.

I never tried to keep him quiet. My husband liked to hear him too.

(17) *Games, Songs, Stories*

As soon as he was on his feet, we started all sorts of games with him (Ring-a-Roses, Baby Bunting, Pat-a-Cake, This Little Piggy, My Daddy Bought Me a Nice New Coat, Ride-a-Cock-Horse, This is the Way a Gentleman Rides). At eighteen months he had a rocking-horse and I made up a poem and a tune for it:

'Dandy-dick, dandy-dick,
Can you go high, can you go quick'.

He was quite fearless on his rocking-horse, and seems much more timid about heights now.

I allowed older children to play with him after about eighteen months, but always with supervision. I remember I wouldn't let a girl of eleven years wheel his pram.

We had a carry-cot till he was about three months, and never carried him in our arms. My husband and I and our relatives on both sides took him out in the pram, usually on Sunday. I didn't take him shopping with me, but left the pram outside my sister's house. Mostly we went to the parks and for different walks. There wasn't much visiting while he was in his pram. I bought him a drop-end pram at one year and two months.

He travelled quite often in a car, in my arms, after four months.

He began to travel in trains, trams and buses at about two.

His first songs were 'Baby Bunting' and 'Little Boy Blue', sung to my own tunes. Then there was a Jewish song 'A Nice Little Wife', which we would sing to him imitating my father's foreign accent. Others were 'Sing a Song of Sixpence', 'Little Fat Doctor', 'Little Polly had a Sister'. We didn't play any instruments specially for him.

We started telling him stories at about one year. The first ones were 'Three Bears' and a censored version of 'Little Red Riding Hood'. My husband made up a lot of his own stories, too. At eighteen months we started reading him stories from a nursery-rhyme book. The usual story-time was just before he went to bed.

His first pictures were in a rag-book of soldiers, trains and so on. We had this before eighteen months.

During his second year he loved playing with a screwdriver, hammers, old plugs and bobbins. Mainly he played by himself, on his own initiative, and didn't make much suggestion of the adults' playing with him.

He had a play-pen from about seven months to a year, but only spent about half an hour a day in it.

He didn't go to parties before he was two—I didn't think it was neccessary at that age.

The songs and the music were about the same in his second year. He began to ask for songs like 'Little Boy Blue' and 'A Nice Little Wife'.